The Airway and Exercise

Editors

J. TOD OLIN
JAMES H. HULL

IMMUNOLOGY AND ALLERGY CLINICS OF NORTH AMERICA

www.immunology.theclinics.com

Consulting Editor
STEPHEN A. TILLES

May 2018 • Volume 38 • Number 2

ELSEVIER

1600 John F. Kennedy Boulevard • Suite 1800 • Philadelphia, Pennsylvania, 19103-2899

http://www.theclinics.com

IMMUNOLOGY AND ALLERGY CLINICS OF NORTH AMERICA Volume 38, Number 2

May 2018 ISSN 0889-8561, ISBN-13: 978-0-323-58358-9

Editor: Jessica McCool

Developmental Editor: Kristen Helm

Immunology and Allergy Clinics of North America (ISSN 0889–8561) is published quarterly by Elsevier Inc., 360 Park Avenue South, New York, NY 10010-1710. Months of issue are February, May, August, and November. Periodicals postage paid at New York, NY and additional mailing offices. Subscription prices are $333.00 per year for US individuals, $565.00 per year for US institutions, $100.00 per year for US students and residents, $411.00 per year for Canadian individuals, $220.00 per year for Canadian students, $717.00 per year for Canadian institutions, $445.00 per year for international individuals, $717.00 per year for international institutions, $220.00 per year for international students. To receive student/resident rate, orders must be accompanied by name of affiliated institution, date of term, and the *signature* of program/residency coordinator on institution letterhead. Orders will be billed at individual rate until proof of status is received. Foreign air speed delivery is included in all *Clinics* subscription prices. All prices are subject to change without notice. **POSTMASTER:** Send address changes to *Immunology and Allergy Clinics of North America*, Elsevier Health Sciences Division, Subscription Customer Service, 3251 Riverport Lane, Maryland Heights, MO 63043. **Customer Service: 1-800-654-2452 (U.S. and Canada); 314-447-8871 (outside U.S. and Canada). Fax: 314-447-8029. E-mail: journalscustomerservice-usa@elsevier.com (for print support); journalsonlinesupport-usa@elsevier.com (for online support).**

Reprints. For copies of 100 or more, of articles in this publication, please contact the Commercial Reprints Department, Elsevier Inc., 360 Park Avenue South, New York, New York 10010-1710. Tel. 212-633-3874, Fax: 212-633-3820, E-mail: reprints@elsevier.com.

Immunology and Allergy Clinics of North America is covered in MEDLINE/PubMed (Index Medicus), Current Contents/Life Sciences, Science Citation Index, ISI/BIOMED, Chemical Abstracts, and EMBASE/Excerpta Medica.

Contributors

CONSULTING EDITOR

STEPHEN A. TILLES, MD
Executive Director, ASTHMA Inc. Clinical Research Center, Partner, Northwest Asthma & Allergy Center, Clinical Professor of Medicine, University of Washington, Seattle, Washington, USA

EDITORS

J. TOD OLIN, MD, MSCS
Director, Pediatric Exercise Tolerance Center, Assistant Professor, Department of Pediatrics, Division of Pediatric Pulmonology, National Jewish Health, Denver, Colorado, USA

JAMES H. HULL, FRCP, PhD
Consultant Respiratory Physician, Honorary Senior Lecturer, Imperial College London, Department of Respiratory Medicine, Royal Brompton & Harefield Hospitals, London, United Kingdom

AUTHORS

ISRAEL AMIRAV, MD
Department of Paediatrics, University of Alberta, Edmonton, Canada

SANDRA D. ANDERSON, PhD, DSc, MD (Hon)
Clinical Professor, Central Clinical School, Sydney Medical School, The University of Sydney, Sydney, New South Wales, Australia

VIBEKE BACKER, MD, DMSci
Professor, Chief Respiratory Physician, Department of Respiratory Medicine, Bispebjerg Hospital, University of Copenhagen, Copenhagen NV, Denmark

J. ANDREW BIRD, MD
Associate Professor, Departments of Pediatrics and Internal Medicine, Division of Allergy and Immunology, University of Texas Southwestern Medical Center, Dallas, Texas, USA

MATTEO BONINI, MD, PhD
Senior Research Fellow, National Heart and Lung Institute (NHLI), Royal Brompton & Harefield Hospitals, Imperial College London, United Kingdom

VALÉRIE BOUGAULT, PhD
Assistant Professor in Physiology, Pluridisciplinary Research Unit Sport, University of Lille, Health Society (URePSSS), Lille, France

JOHN D. BRANNAN, PhD
Scientific Director, Department of Respiratory and Sleep Medicine, John Hunter Hospital, New Lambton, New South Wales, Australia

DOMINIQUE M. BULLENS, MD, PhD
Paediatric Immunology, Department of Microbiology and Immunology, KU Leuven, Clinical Department of Pediatrics, University Hospitals Leuven, Leuven, Belgium

JOHN DICKINSON, PhD
School of Sport and Exercise Sciences, University of Kent, United Kingdom

JEMMA HAINES, BSc (Hons), CertMRCSLT
Consultant Speech and Language Therapist, Respiratory Medicine Department, University Hospital of South Manchester, NHS Foundation Trust, North West Lung Centre, Manchester, United Kingdom

TEAL S. HALLSTRAND, MD, MPH
Associate Professor, Department of Medicine, Division of Pulmonary, Critical Care and Sleep Medicine, Center for Lung Biology, University of Washington, Seattle, Washington, USA

THOMAS HALVORSEN, MD, PhD
Department of Paediatrics, Haukeland University Hospital, Department of Clinical Science, Section for Paediatrics, University of Bergen, Bergen, Norway

JOHN-HELGE HEIMDAL, MD, PhD
Chairman, Department of Surgery, Associate Professor, Department of Otorhinolaryngology, Head and Neck Surgery, Haukeland University Hospital, Bergen University, Bergen, Norway

PETER W. HELLINGS, MD, PhD
Laboratory of Clinical Immunology, Department of Microbiology and Immunology, KU Leuven, Clinical Department of Otorhinolaryngology, Head and Neck Surgery, University Hospitals Leuven, UZ Leuven, Leuven, Belgium

MORTEN HOSTRUP, PhD
Department of Nutrition, Exercise and Sports, University of Copenhagen, Department of Respiratory Medicine, Bispebjerg University Hospital, Copenhagen, Denmark

VALERIE HOX, MD, PhD
Division of Otorhinolaryngology, Cliniques Universitaires Saint-Luc, Brussels, Belgium

JAMES H. HULL, FRCP, PhD
Consultant Respiratory Physician, Honorary Senior Lecturer, Imperial College London, Department of Respiratory Medicine, Royal Brompton & Harefield Hospitals, London, United Kingdom

PASCALE KIPPELEN, PhD
Senior Lecturer, Department of Life Sciences, Division of Sport, Health and Exercise Sciences, Centre for Human Performance, Exercise and Rehabilitation, Brunel University London, Uxbridge, United Kingdom

JULIANA K. LITTS, MA, CCC-SLP
Instructor, Faculty and Speech-Language Pathologist, Department of Otolaryngology, University of Colorado Hospital, Aurora, Colorado, USA

ROBERT MAAT, MD, PhD
Senior Consultant, Department of Otolaryngology, Röpcke-Zweers Hospital, Hardenberg, The Netherlands

JOHN MASTRONARDE, MD, MSc
Chair, Department of Medical Education, Providence Portland Medical Center, Professor, Pulmonary/Critical Care Medicine, Oregon Health & Science University, Portland, Oregon, USA

CAMERON W. McLAUGHLIN, DO, Capt, USAF, MC
Fellow, Pulmonary/Critical Care Service (MCHE-ZMD-P), Department of Medicine, San Antonio Military Medical Center, JBSA Fort Sam Houston, Texas, USA

MICHAEL J. MORRIS, MD
Faculty, Pulmonary/Critical Care Service (MCHE-ZMD-P), Department of Medicine, San Antonio Military Medical Center, JBSA Fort Sam Houston, Texas, USA

EMILY NAUMAN, MA, CCC-SLP
Speech-Language Pathologist, Rehab Department, National Jewish Health, Denver, Colorado, USA

LEIF NORDANG, MD, PhD
Associate Professor, Department of Surgical Sciences, Otorhinolaryngology and Head and Neck Surgery, Uppsala University, Uppsala, Sweden

KATARINA NORLANDER, MD, PhD
Department of Surgical Sciences, Otorhinolaryngology and Head and Neck Surgery, Uppsala University, Uppsala, Sweden

J. TOD OLIN, MD, MSCS
Director, Pediatric Exercise Tolerance Center, Assistant Professor, Department of Pediatrics, Division of Pediatric Pulmonology, National Jewish Health, Denver, Colorado, USA

CELESTE PORSBJERG, MD, PhD
Associate Clinical Research Professor, Respiratory Research Unit, Department of Respiratory Medicine, Bispebjerg University Hospital, Copenhagen NV, Denmark

OLA DRANGE RØKSUND, DPT, PhD
Faculty of Health and Social Sciences, Western Norway University of Applied Sciences, Department of Paediatrics, Haukeland University Hospital, Bergen, Norway

KENNETH W. RUNDELL, PhD, FACSM
Adjunct Associate Professor, Department of Basic Sciences, Geisinger Commonwealth School of Medicine, Scranton, Pennsylvania, USA

SVEN F. SEYS, PhD
Laboratory of Clinical immunology, Department of Microbiology and Immunology, KU Leuven, Leuven, Belgium

MONICA SHAFFER, MA, CCC-SLP
Speech-Language Pathologist, Rehab Department, National Jewish Health, Denver, Colorado, USA

WILLIAM SILVERS, MD
Clinical Professor of Medicine, University of Colorado School of Medicine, Denver, Colorado, USA

JAMES M. SMOLIGA, DVM, PhD, FACSM
Assistant Professor in Physiology, Department of Physical Therapy, High Point University, High Point, North Carolina, USA

BRECHT STEELANT, PhD
Laboratory of Clinical Immunology, Department of Microbiology and Immunology,
KU Leuven, Leuven, Belgium

EMIL SCHWARZ WALSTED, MD, PhD
Respiratory Research Unit, Department of Respiratory Medicine, Bispebjerg University
Hospital, Copenhagen, Denmark

ERIKA WESTHOFF (CARLSON), MA, CC-AASP
Erika Westhoff Performance, Pleasanton, Colorado, USA

JEFFREY T. WOODS, MD, MC, USA
Fellow, Pulmonary/Critical Care Service (MCHE-ZMD-P), Department of Medicine,
San Antonio Military Medical Center, JBSA Fort Sam Houston, Texas, USA

Contents

> Exercise is a common trigger of bronchoconstriction. In recent years, there has been an increased understanding of the pathophysiology of exercise-induced bronchoconstriction. Although evaporative water loss and thermal changes have been recognized as stimuli for exercise-induced bronchoconstriction, accumulating evidence points toward a pivotal role for the airway epithelium in orchestrating the inflammatory response linked to exercise-induced bronchoconstriction. Overproduction of inflammatory mediators, underproduction of protective lipid mediators, and infiltration of the airways with eosinophils and mast cells are all established contributors to exercise-induced bronchoconstriction. Sensory nerve activation and release of neuropeptides may be important in exercise-induced bronchoconstriction, but further research is warranted.

> An association between airway dysfunction and airborne pollutant inhalation exists. Volatilized airborne fluorocarbons in ski wax rooms, particulate matter, and trichloromines in indoor environments are suspect to high prevalence of exercise-induced bronchoconstriction and new-onset asthma in athletes competing in cross-country skiing, ice rink sports, and swimming. Ozone is implicated in acute decreases in lung function and the development of new-onset asthma from exposure during exercise. Mechanisms and genetic links are proposed for pollution-related new-onset asthma. Oxidative stress from airborne pollutant inhalation is a common thread to progression of airway damage. Key pollutants and mechanisms for each are discussed.

> The transient airway narrowing that occurs as a result of exercise is defined as exercise-induced bronchoconstriction (EIB). The prevalence of EIB has been reported to be up to 90% in asthmatic patients, reflecting the level of disease control. However, EIB may develop even in subjects without clinical asthma, particularly in children, athletes, and

patients with atopy or rhinitis and following respiratory infections. The intensity, duration, and type of training have been associated with the occurrence of EIB. In athletes, EIB seems to be only partly reversible, and exercise seems to be a causative factor of airway inflammation and symptoms.

Exercise-induced bronchoconstriction (EIB) is a form of airway hyperresponsiveness that occurs with or without current symptoms of asthma. EIB is an indicator of active and treatable pathophysiology in persons with asthma. The objective documentation of EIB permits the identification of an individual who may be at risk during a recreational sporting activity or when exercising as an occupational duty. EIB can be identified with laboratory exercise testing or surrogate tests for EIB. These tests include eucapnic voluntary hyperpnea and osmotic stimuli (eg, inhaled mannitol) and offer improved diagnostic sensitivity to identify EIB and improved standardization when compared with laboratory exercise.

Exercise-induced bronchoconstriction (EIB) is the transient narrowing of the airways during and after exercise that occurs in response to increased ventilation in susceptible individuals. It occurs across the age spectrum in patients with underlying asthma and can occur in athletes without baseline asthma. The inflammatory mechanisms underlying EIB in patients without asthma may be distinct from those underlying EIB in patients with asthma. This article summarizes mechanistic and clinical data that can guide the choice of chronic and acute pharmacologic therapies targeting the control of EIB. Relevant regulations from the World Anti-Doping Agency are also discussed.

Pharmacologic management of exercise-induced bronchoconstriction (EIB) is the mainstay of preventative therapy. There are some nonpharmacologic interventions, however, that may assist the management of EIB. This article discusses these nonpharmacologic interventions and how they may be applied to patients and athletes with EIB.

Physical exercise requires proper function of the upper and lower airways to meet exertional ventilatory requirements. Athletes performing frequent intensive exercise experience more sinonasal symptoms and demonstrate objective decreases in sinonasal function when compared with the general population. Sinonasal dysfunction is known to interfere with sport performance. Nasal epithelial injury, neutrophilic influx, and decreased mucociliary clearance have been associated with intensive training. In this article, the authors provide a comprehensive overview of the prevalence of sinonasal disease in athletes, the possible underlying pathophysiologic mechanisms, and a summary of diagnostic and treatment options.

Exertional dyspnea is common in health and disease. Despite having known for centuries that breathlessness can arise from the larynx, exercise-induced laryngeal obstruction is a more prevalent condition than previously assumed. This article provides a brief overview of the history, epidemiology, and pathophysiology of exercise-induced laryngeal obstruction.

Exertional dyspnea can be a manifestation of dysfunction in a variety of organ systems. Exercise-induced laryngeal obstruction (EILO), a condition previously known as vocal cord dysfunction and paradoxic vocal fold motion, is defined as inappropriate, reversible narrowing of the larynx during vigorous exercise. EILO is usually characterized by typical symptoms, which nevertheless frequently are confused with those of other conditions, including asthma. Laryngoscopy performed as symptoms evolve from rest to peak exercise is pivotal in patient workup. Moving forward, laryngoscopy findings that definitively characterize EILO need to be defined as do objective measures that can quantitate absolute laryngeal measurements during exercise.

Exercise-induced laryngeal obstruction is a condition that restricts respiration during exercise via inappropriate glottic or supraglottic obstruction. The literature supports behavioral treatment provided by a speech-language pathologist as an effective means of treating exercise-induced laryngeal obstruction. Treatment includes educating the patient, training on relaxation, instruction on paced exercise, and use of various breathing techniques to optimize laryngeal aperture. Intervention for patients with exercise-induced laryngeal obstruction may be delivered by a speech-language pathologist, given their clinical skill of facilitating long-term behavioral change and expertise in the laryngeal mechanism.

Exercise-induced laryngeal obstruction causes severe shortness of breath during exercise. Episodes are associated with severe distress. These patients and those with inducible laryngeal obstruction triggered by other factors have been noted to demonstrate mental health disorders, personality features that may be associated with symptoms, and dysfunctional stress responses. This literature review calls attention to the observation that patients with isolated exercise-induced laryngeal obstruction are generally mentally healthy. The authors review available metrics to assess traits and stress responses in performance psychology. They also discuss a therapeutic performance psychology framework.

 Video content accompanies this article at http://www.immunology. theclinics.com.

Respiratory distress during exercise can be caused by exercise-induced laryngeal obstruction (EILO). The obstruction may appear at the level of the laryngeal inlet (supraglottic), similar to supraglottic collapse observed in infants with congenital laryngomalacia (CLM). This observation has encouraged surgeons to treat supraglottic EILO with procedures proven efficient for severe CLM. This article summarizes key features of the published experience related to surgical treatment of EILO. Supraglottoplasty is an irreversible procedure with potential complications. Surgery should be restricted to cases where the supraglottic laryngeal obstruction significantly affects the quality of life in patients for whom conservative treatment modalities have failed.

Excessive dynamic airway collapse is a relatively new diagnosis separate from tracheobronchomalacia that is manifested by functional collapse of the large airways. This condition is most commonly described in patients with underlying obstructive lung disease, such as chronic obstructive pulmonary disease and asthma, and may contribute to increased dyspnea, cough, or exacerbations. There are few data published on the role of excessive dynamic airway collapse as related specifically to exercise. It was recently described as the cause for exertional dyspnea in individuals without underlying lung disease.

Exercise is increasingly viewed as a preventative and therapeutic modality for medical and behavioral health disorders. Therefore, it is imperative that the medical and scientific communities minimize barriers that discourage exercise. This issue of *Immunology and Allergy Clinics of North America* details a "total airway approach" to the evaluation of exertional respiratory problems. Reviews guide clinicians through evaluation and therapy. Moving forward, there is much room for growth with respect to research in each of these areas as well as for common inflammatory pathways and neurophysiologic coupling across all airway segments.

Food allergy should be suspected in individuals with a history of immediate reactivity following ingestion (ie, typically within 20 minutes and almost always within 2 hours) with typical symptoms of immunoglobulin E–mediated reactivity (eg, urticaria, angioedema, coughing, wheezing, vomiting). Testing for food allergy should focus on the most likely allergen to provoke the reaction based on the patient's history. Safe introduction of peanut-containing foods into the diet of an infant at high risk of developing peanut allergy at 4 to 6 months is likely to reduce the risk of peanut allergy.

IMMUNOLOGY AND ALLERGY CLINICS OF NORTH AMERICA

FORTHCOMING ISSUES

August 2018
Mastocytosis
Mariana C. Castells, *Editor*

November 2018
Biomarkers in Allergy and Asthma
Flavia Hoyte and Rohit K. Katial, *Editors*

February 2019
Primary Immune Deficiencies
Lisa Kobrynski, *Editor*

RECENT ISSUES

February 2018
Food Allergy
J. Andrew Bird, *Editor*

November 2017
Drug Hypersensitivity and Desensitizations
Mariana C. Castells, *Editor*

August 2017
Angioedema
Marc A. Riedl, *Editor*

ISSUE OF RELATED INTEREST

Emergency Medicine Clinics of North America, February 2016 (Vol. 34, No. 1)
Respiratory Emergencies
Robert J. Vissers and Michael A. Gibbs, *Editors*
Available at: http://www.emed.theclinics.com/

THE CLINICS ARE AVAILABLE ONLINE!
Access your subscription at:
www.theclinics.com

Foreword

Exercise-Induced Airway Dysfunction in Athletes

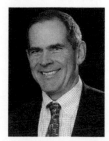

Stephen A. Tilles, MD
Consulting Editor

In recent decades, exercise-induced dysfunction of the airways has become a common presenting complaint in the office practices of both asthma specialists and primary care providers. Part of this growing unmet need appears to be due to exercise-induced bronchospasm (EIB), and although the recognition that exercise is a common trigger of asthma symptoms is not new, EIB in athletes appears to be more common than previously appreciated. In fact, there is a growing consensus that EIB involves mediator release from inflammatory cells in the airway, even in patients who do not otherwise have clinical asthma. Indeed, it can be argued that EIB has become an occupational disease.

The upper airway is also vulnerable as a source of exercise-induced symptoms, particularly when there is paradoxical adduction of the larynx resulting in dyspnea and other symptoms. Exercise-induced vocal cord dysfunction (VCD), also known as "exercise-induced laryngeal obstruction" (EILO), is often confused with EIB and is a leading cause of exercise-induced dyspnea in both competitive and elite athletes. Contrary to assertions of early case series authors, exercise-induced VCD is not a manifestation of anxiety, but in fact affects a wide spectrum of athletes, particularly adolescent women. Without the benefit of animal models, large-scale controlled clinical trials, or even agreed upon pathology, our understanding of exercise-induced VCD/EILO largely stems from anecdotal case series and therefore presents a desperate need for collaborative investigation to better understand how to diagnose, treat, and possibly prevent this disorder.

In this issue of *Immunology and Allergy Clinics of North America*, J Tod Olin and James H. Hull have thoughtfully assembled a comprehensive range of scholarly scientific and clinical reviews relevant to exercise-induced airway disorders. These articles focus on clinically relevant topics, such as diagnostic testing, management strategies, as well as relevant comorbidities. This outstanding *Immunology and Allergy Clinics of*

Immunol Allergy Clin N Am 38 (2018) xiii–xiv
https://doi.org/10.1016/j.iac.2018.02.002
0889-8561/18/© 2018 Published by Elsevier Inc.

North America issue is an essential up-to-date reference and will be of interest to specialists in allergy, pulmonary, sports medicine, and primary care.

Stephen A. Tilles, MD
ASTHMA Inc. Clinical Research Center
Northwest Asthma and Allergy Center
University of Washington, 9725 3rd Avenue Northeast, Suite 500
Seattle, WA 98115, USA

E-mail address:
stilles@nwasthma.com

Preface

Exercise and the Total Airway: A Call to Action

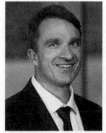 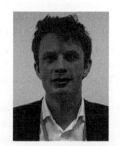

J. Tod Olin, MD, MSCS   James H. Hull, FRCP, PhD
Editors

> *The condition of exercise is not a mere variant of the condition of rest, it is the essence of the machine.*
>
> —*Sir John Bancroft*

Exercise is a fundamental part of human existence, and yet it is now well recognized that strenuous exercise places significant stress on the respiratory system and airway tract specifically. Indeed, while mild to moderate exercise is generally accepted as being beneficial for respiratory health, strenuous exercise, especially when performed very frequently and in noxious environments, is associated with a considerable degree of chemical, mechanical, and thermal stress for the airway tract.[1]

It is therefore not surprising that airway-focused respiratory symptoms (eg, cough, wheeze, and excessive mucus production) and their associated morbidity (eg, respiratory tract infection) are highly prevalent in athletic individuals.[2] Indeed, troublesome respiratory symptoms represent the most common noninjury reason for athletes to consult a physician, and asthma is now recognized to be the most prevalent chronic medical condition in Olympians.[3] Moreover, when respiratory symptoms occur in competitive athletes, they have not only an immediate impact on health and quality of life but also an obvious and deleterious impact on ability to perform and compete.[4] The same symptoms are also important to individuals of all athletic levels and may be a deterrent to exercising for some.

It is for this reason that this special issue of the *Immunology and Allergy Clinics of North America* has been devoted to airway dysfunction and exercise in athletic individuals. The issue could be viewed as a revision of the successful and similarly themed issue of 2013 (edited by Professor Sandra D. Anderson, http://www.immunology.theclinics.com/issue/S0889-8561(13)X0003-7); however, there are several important

Immunol Allergy Clin N Am 38 (2018) xv–xix
https://doi.org/10.1016/j.iac.2018.02.001
0889-8561/18/© 2018 Published by Elsevier Inc.   immunology.theclinics.com

and notable differences. Certainly, over the past five years there is growing appreciation that any consideration of the airway in exercise shouldn't simply be confined to the lower airways. From both a clinical and a basic science perspective, it is logical to consider the contribution from both the upper, laryngeal section and the central components of the airway.[5] Indeed an understanding of how the entire airway is impacted and functions during exercise in athletic individuals is fundamental to progress our understanding and certainly important to help clinicians provide the best treatment to individuals presenting with exercise-associated respiratory symptoms. The discussion below and articles in this issue endorse this view, and yet currently many clinicians appear to overlook the role of the nasal and laryngeal dysfunction in the development of exertional respiratory symptoms. This issue of the *Immunology and Allergy Clinics of North America*, therefore, for the first time, acts to improve the understanding and appreciation of the "total" airway in causing respiratory dysfunction in athletic individuals.

In order to achieve this aim, we have assembled and invited leading authorities in their respective fields to contribute and to outline the respective importance of the various sections of the airway tract. The content of this issue thus aims to provide an overview of the current state of knowledge from the "tip of the nose to the smallest airways."

Since the last similarly themed special issue in the *Immunology and Allergy Clinics of North America*, our understanding of the factors driving the development of exercise-induced bronchoconstriction (EIB) in endurance athletes has evolved, with growing appreciation that both epithelial damage and neuronal (hyper-) sensitivity are likely to be relevant in the pathogenesis of EIB and its clinical manifestations.[6,7] Environmental and noxious atmospheric exposure is key in these processes, and any consideration of the factors driving airway symptoms cannot discount these interactions in competitive athletic individuals, who spend prolonged periods "exposed" in both training and competition situations.[8] These areas are therefore covered, in detail, in several articles on EIB, covering mechanisms and biomarkers (in the article by Drs Kippelen, Anderson, and Hallstrand) and the impact of environment on the airway (in the article by Drs Rundell, Smoliga, and Bougault).

Certainly sport-related asthma has evolved to have a big impact on the global media stage. Treatment, antidoping considerations, and competitive advantage are all closely intertwined and command significant media attention in this context. Accordingly, it is vital that the diagnosis of EIB is robust and that all treatment avenues (eg, including nonpharmaceutical options) are explored in treating afflicted individuals. Again, this issue of the *Immunology and Allergy Clinics of North America* provides authoritative background overview of EIB (in the article by Drs Bonini and Silvers), an article focused on how to best diagnose this condition (written by Drs Brannan and Porsbjerg), and articles on how best to approach both the pharmacologic (written by Drs Backer and Mastronarde) and nonpharmacologic treatment (written by Drs Dickinson, Amirav, and Hostrup).

This special issue of the *Immunology and Allergy Clinics of North America* also builds on that published in the previous issue. In this respect, for years, clinicians managing asthma have understood that effective and comprehensive management of asthma is dependent on consideration and optimal management of all components of the airway. Indeed a "systematic assessment process" underpins high-quality care in difficult-to-treat asthma.[9] Accordingly, optimal care in severe asthma relies on consideration and treatment of comorbid factors, and for instance, treatment of nasal disease, laryngeal disease, dysfunctional breathing, and gastroesophageal reflux.[10] This approach doesn't necessarily mandate subscription to the view of a "unified airway hypothesis[11]"; however, in the context of vigorous exercise, the entire airway tract is exposed to the "stimulus," and thus to consider EIB alone discounts the potentially important role of the other key components of the airway on symptom genesis.

In athletic individuals, normal upper airway function is vitally important both at rest and during exercise. The nasal passage acts to filter environmental toxins and allergens, to humidify and modulate air temperature, and to provide a brake-type function on airway resistance. Clinically, optimizing nasal function is central in order to facilitate improved breathing patterns and potentially to reduce frequency of upper-respiratory tract infection. Yet there remain a number of unanswered questions regarding the interaction between the nasal passage and lower airways (eg, how inflammation co-exists/interacts) to modulate overall function. These issues are reviewed and covered in the article written by Drs Steelant, Hox, Hellings, Bullens, and Seys, with clinical sections specific to athlete care.

A key and evolving field is focused on the appreciation that, for many young athletic individuals, closure of the laryngeal inlet may be the factor underpinning their dyspnea and wheeze. Exercise-associated vocal cord dysfunction has been recognized for over 30 years; however, it is only within the past five years that there has been a groundswell of interest in understanding the role of the larynx during exercise and specifically exercise-induced laryngeal obstruction (EILO).[12] Multiple terms have been used to describe this entity over this time, and although the concept of vocal cord dysfunction and parodoxic vocal fold motion analysis remains relevant in the context of exercise, they appear to inadequately capture the true nature of the physiologic abnormality that occurs (ie, it is now evident that it is additional laryngeal structures [eg, arytenoids] that are very relevant in causing glottic closure).[13] Work in the last two years reveals that EILO may explain exercise-associated dyspnea in as many as 1 in 10 adolescents and certainly appears to be the key differential diagnosis for EIB in young athletes.[14,15] Robust diagnosis of EILO mandates objective testing, and the continuous laryngoscopy during exercise test is now the de facto gold standard.[16] This test modality has evolved significantly and can now be applied in a number of sport-specific settings (eg, swimming[17] and rowing[18]) to successfully provide biofeedback.[19] A comprehensive overview of the background (addressed by Drs Nordang, Norlander, and Walsted) and diagnostic approach (addressed by Drs Røksund, Olin, and Halvorsen) in EILO is provided in this issue of the *Immunology and Allergy Clinics of North America.*

Intervention studies in EILO are currently limited, and indeed, there are no published randomized controlled trials. This acknowledged, there have been a number of case-control and retrospective analyses forwarding the role of both therapy-based (in the article by Drs Bergevin, Litts, Nauman, and Haines) and psychological treatment (in the article by Drs Olin and Westhoff) and indeed surgical intervention (in the article by Drs Heimdal, Maat, and Nordang). Again, leaders in the field provide an overview of these areas.

Finally, the airway tract has sections that are often simply viewed as having "conduit" function. The large/central airways are often viewed in this way; however, there is now a growing appreciation of the fact that the trachea and main bronchi may actually impact ventilatory function, and certainly excessive dynamic airways closure is described as causing respiratory symptoms in some athletic individuals.[20] It may also be that this section of the airway "interacts" with the upper airway and is potentially relevant in modulating ventilatory dynamics and lung emptying.[21] The article by Drs Morris, Woods, and McLaughlin provides an overview of the current state of knowledge in this area.

A key challenge moving forward is how best to engage clinicians in considering the various subsections of the airway and their potential contribution to the development of exertional respiratory symptoms. EILO is frequently overlooked with data, indicating a significant delay to diagnosis with misdiagnosis and subsequent mistreatment as asthma.[22] Certainly more needs to be done to highlight the importance of considering all aspects of the airway tract, when a clinician is reviewing a young athletic individual wIth airway-centric symptoms. It is with these factors borne in mind that this publication of the *Immunology and Allergy Clinics of North America* is welcomed, and we encourage any scientist and/or clinician with an interest or investment in this area to digest and absorb all articles and to consider the "total airway" in their future practice. Only then can we can consider this a true call to action, to ensure individuals enjoy and participate in what is the "essence of the machine" and without respiratory dysfunction.

J. Tod Olin, MD, MSCS
Pediatric Exercise Tolerance Center
Department of Pediatrics
Division of Pediatric Pulmonology
National Jewish Health
1400 Jackson Street
Denver, CO 80206, USA

James H. Hull, FRCP, PhD
Royal Brompton Hospital
Imperial College
Department of Respiratory Medicine
Royal Brompton Hospital, Fulham Road
London SW3 6HP, UK

E-mail addresses:
OlinT@NJHealth.org (J.T. Olin)
j.hull@rbht.nhs.uk (J.H. Hull)

REFERENCES

1. Anderson SD, Kippelen P. Airway injury as a mechanism for exercise-induced bronchoconstriction in elite athletes. J Allergy Clin Immunol 2008; 122:225–35.
2. Hull JH, Ansley L, Robson-Ansley P, et al. Managing respiratory problems in athletes. Clin Med (Lond) 2012;12:351–6.
3. Fitch KD. An overview of asthma and airway hyper-responsiveness in Olympic athletes. Br J Sports Med 2012;46(6):413–6.
4. Price OJ, Hull JH. Asthma in elite athletes: who cares? Clin Pulmon Med 2014; 21(2):68–75.
5. Bardin PG, Johnston SL, Hamilton G. Middle airway obstruction—it may be happening under our noses. Thorax 2013;68:396–8.
6. Couto M, Kurowski M, Moreira A, et al. Mechanisms of exercise-induced bronchoconstriction in athletes: current perspectives and future challenges. Allergy 2018;73(1):8–16.
7. Belvisi MG, Birrell MA, Khalid S, et al. Neurophenotypes in airway diseases. Insights from translational cough studies. Am J Respir Crit Care Med 2016;193: 1364–72.

8. Price OJ, Ansley L, Menzies-Gow A, et al. Airway dysfunction in elite athletes—an occupational lung disease? Allergy 2013;68:1343–52.
9. Gibeon D, Heaney LG, Brightling CE, et al. Dedicated severe asthma services improve health-care use and quality of life. Chest 2015;148:870–6.
10. Porsbjerg C, Menzies-Gow A. Co-morbidities in severe asthma: clinical impact and management. Respirology 2017;22:651–61.
11. Nayak AS. A common pathway: asthma and allergic rhinitis. Allergy Asthma Proc 2002;23:359–65.
12. Olin JT, Clary MS, Deardorff EH, et al. Inducible laryngeal obstruction during exercise: moving beyond vocal cords with new insights. Phys Sportsmed 2015;43:13–21.
13. Maat RC, Røksund OD, Halvorsen T, et al. Audiovisual assessment of exercise-induced laryngeal obstruction: reliability and validity of observations. Eur Arch Otorhinolaryngol 2009;266:1929–36.
14. Johansson H, Norlander K, Berglund L, et al. Prevalence of exercise-induced bronchoconstriction and exercise-induced laryngeal obstruction in a general adolescent population. Thorax 2015;70:57–63.
15. Walsted NE, Hull JH, Backer V. High prevalence of exercise-induced laryngeal obstruction in athletes. Med Sci Sports Exerc 2013;45(11):2030–5.
16. Heimdal J-H, Roksund OD, Halvorsen T, et al. Continuous laryngoscopy exercise test: a method for visualizing laryngeal dysfunction during exercise. Laryngoscope 2006;116:52–7.
17. Walsted ES, Swanton LL, van van Someren K, et al. Laryngoscopy during swimming: a novel diagnostic technique to characterize swimming-induced laryngeal obstruction. Laryngoscope 2017;127(10):2298–301.
18. Panchasara B, Nelson C, Niven R, et al. Lesson of the month: rowing-induced laryngeal obstruction: a novel cause of exertional dyspnoea: characterised by direct laryngoscopy. Thorax 2015;70(1):95–7.
19. Olin JT, Deardorff EH, Fan EM, et al. Therapeutic laryngoscopy during exercise: a novel non-surgical therapy for refractory EILO. Pediatr Pulmonol 2017;52:813–9.
20. Weinstein DJ, Hull JE, Ritchie BL, et al. Exercise-associated excessive dynamic airway collapse in military personnel. Ann Am Thorac Soc 2016;13:1476–82.
21. Baz M, Haji GS, Menzies-Gow A, et al. Dynamic laryngeal narrowing during exercise: a mechanism for generating intrinsic PEEP in COPD? Thorax 2015;70(3):251–7.
22. Hall A, Thomas M, Sandhu G, et al. Exercise-induced laryngeal obstruction: a common and overlooked cause of exertional breathlessness. Br J Gen Pract 2016;66:e683–5.

Mechanisms and Biomarkers of Exercise-Induced Bronchoconstriction

Pascale Kippelen, PhD[a], Sandra D. Anderson, PhD, DSc[b],*,
Teal S. Hallstrand, MD, MPH[c]

KEYWORDS

- Hyperpnea • Water loss • Osmolarity • Epithelium • Mast cells • Eosinophils
- Eicosanoids • Sensory nerves

KEY POINTS

- The conditioning of inhaled air during exercise-hyperpnea initiates osmotic and vascular events that lead, in susceptible individuals, to airway narrowing.
- A loss of physical barrier integrity and impairment in signaling and secretory functions of the airway epithelium increases the susceptibility to exercise-induced bronchoconstriction.
- Airway smooth muscle contraction and mucin release in individuals with exercise-induced bronchoconstriction are mediated predominantly by release of inflammatory mediators with associated activation of neural pathways.
- Cysteinyl leukotrienes and prostaglandin D_2 are the primary inflammatory mediators released into the airways from mast cells and eosinophils during exercise-induced bronchoconstriction.

INTRODUCTION

The underlying basis for exercise-induced bronchoconstriction (EIB) is becoming increasingly understood. Initial work starting in the 1970s revealed the major determinants of EIB in susceptible individuals. The aims of this review are to examine the respective roles of evaporative water loss and thermal changes as stimuli to EIB;

Disclosure Statement: Dr S.D. Anderson is the inventor of the mannitol test used for the diagnosis of bronchial hyperresponsiveness and receives a share of the royalties from the sale of Aridol and Osmohale paid to Royal Prince Alfred Hospital by Pharmaxis Ltd. Drs P. Kippelen and T.S. Hallstrand have no conflict of interest.
[a] Department of Life Sciences, Division of Sport, Health and Exercise Sciences, Centre for Human Performance, Exercise and Rehabilitation, Brunel University London, Kingston Lane, Uxbridge UB8 3PH, UK; [b] Central Clinical School, Sydney Medical School, University of Sydney, Parramatta Road, Sydney New South Wales 2006, Australia; [c] Department of Medicine, Division of Pulmonary, Critical Care and Sleep Medicine, Center for Lung Biology, University of Washington, Box 358052, 850 Republican Street, Seattle, WA 98109-4714, USA
* Corresponding author. PO Box 87, Balmain, New South Wales 2041, Australia.
E-mail address: sandra.anderson@sydney.edu.au

Immunol Allergy Clin N Am 38 (2018) 165–182
https://doi.org/10.1016/j.iac.2018.01.008   immunology.theclinics.com
0889-8561/18/© 2018 Elsevier Inc. All rights reserved.

provide evidence that loss of physical barrier functions of the epithelium during exercise-induced hyperpnea is associated with the development of bronchoconstriction in susceptible individuals; discuss the central role of leukocyte activation and the associated generation of lipid mediators and release of neuropeptides that sustain bronchoconstriction during EIB; and consider the role that regional airway closure may play in the development of EIB.

CONDITIONING THE AIR INSPIRED DURING EXERCISE

Under most conditions of exercise, the air inspired needs to be heated and humidified to body conditions ($37°C$, 100% relative humidity, or 44 mg H_2O/L) before it enters the alveoli. As a result, heat and water are lost from the airway surface during inspiration. The number of generations involved in conditioning depends on the level of ventilation reached and sustained during exercise, and the temperature and water content of the inspired air.[1]

Heat Loss as a Stimulus to Airway Narrowing

Cooling of the airways, from heat lost through vaporization of water and from heating the inspired air, was initially identified as a potential stimulus for EIB.[2] The proposal was subsequently extended to include a rewarming of the airways after exercise[3] (**Fig. 1**). This hypothesis suggested that cooling initiated vasoconstriction during exercise, followed by a reactive (or rebound) hyperemia at the end of exercise.[3] These vascular events are most significant when air of subzero temperature is inspired during intense exercise of 4 minutes or more[4] and when the smaller airways are recruited into the conditioning process, but are unlikely to occur in temperate or hot environments. These vascular events may be relevant to anyone performing vigorous exercise in cold conditions and may serve to amplify airway narrowing in individuals with asthma who may have a more rapid and exaggerated vascular response than non-asthmatics.[5,6]

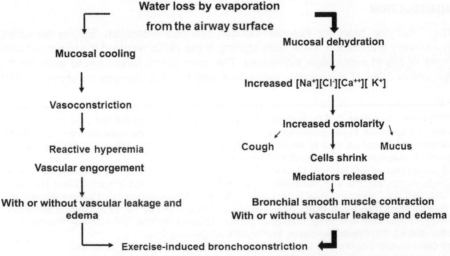

Fig. 1. Both airway cooling and mucosal dehydration occur in response to evaporative water loss from the airway surface. These events lead to exercise-induced bronchoconstriction. (*From* Rundell KW, Anderson SD, Sue-Chu M, et al. Air quality and temperature effects on exercise-induced bronchoconstriction. Compr Physiol 2015;5(2):581; with permission.)

Water Loss as a Stimulus to Airway Narrowing

It is now well-recognized that cooling and rewarming of the airways are not prerequisites for EIB. In individuals with asthma, EIB occurs when hot dry air is inhaled during exercise[7–9] and when the airways are not cooled below their temperature at rest.[10]

The concentration of water in the inspired air is an important determinant of EIB,[11] with the rate of water loss during exercise relating directly to the severity of the airway response in an individual.[12] Importantly, the stimulus to EIB acts at the surface of the airways, because EIB is prevented simply by inhaling fully humidified air at body temperature.[11,13] A loss of water by evaporation, in humidifying large volumes of air in a short time, is thought to cause a transient increase in concentration of ions (eg, Na^+, Cl^-, Ca^{++}) in the airway surface liquid (ASL)[14] (see **Fig. 1**). This osmotic stimulus occurs after intense exercise when dry air of any temperature (cold or hot) is inspired, providing the duration of exercise is sufficient.

Because the surface area of the first 10 generations of airways is 742 cm^2 and contains less than 0.7 mL of ASL,[15,16] only a small loss of water would increase osmolarity above the normal value of approximately 320 to 340 mOsm. A mathematical model, based on in vivo observations,[17] predicted that breathing air of 26°C and 35% relative humidity at 60 L/min would result in a cumulative loss of 0.44 mL per minute from the first 12 generations of airways.[18,19] It is likely that this rate of water loss exceeds the rate of replacement across the epithelium, leading to a transient increase in the osmolarity of the ASL.

Although methodological limitations render the accurate measurement of changes in ASL osmolarity difficult,[20] there is direct evidence for evaporative water loss from the airways involved in conditioning the air. The mucociliary clearance rate was shown to be reduced during hyperpnea with dry air (but not humid air).[21] This reduction, however, occurred more markedly in people with asthma compared with healthy individuals, suggesting that the rate of water movement across the epithelium toward the lumen is slower in populations prone to EIB.[21]

An increase in ion concentration of the ASL during exercise would act as an osmotic stimulus for transport of water to the airway surface from the epithelial cells and other cells on or near the airway surface. Because the basolateral membrane is less permeable to water than the apical membrane, it was proposed that epithelial cells, as well as other cells, would have a reduction in volume.[22] It is the regulatory volume increase after cell volume decrease that is thought to provide the signal for mediator release. The source of water to replace the epithelial cell volume is the submucosa, and small changes in its osmolarity could be the signal to the increase in bronchial blood flow that occurs when breathing dry air.[23–25] The osmotic stimulus to EIB is further supported by evidence that airway narrowing can be provoked in asthmatics by inhalation of hyperosmolar saline.[26] Further, the airway response to hypertonic saline is related to mast cell number (assessed by brush biopsy).[27] Mediators released in response to osmotic challenge with dry powder mannitol[28] are the same as exercise[29] and blocked by the same drugs.[30,31]

The transient increase in osmolarity of the ASL during exercise creates an environment known to be favorable for release of mediators from cells in or near the airway surface (eg, epithelial cells, sensory nerves, mast cells, and eosinophils). Although some mediators (prostaglandin E_2 [PGE_2]) may induce bronchodilation during exercise, other mediators (neurokinins, prostaglandin D_2 [PGD_2], cysteinyl leukotrienes) provoke airway narrowing by acting, either directly on bronchial smooth muscle or via sensory nerves (**Fig. 2**).[29,31,32]

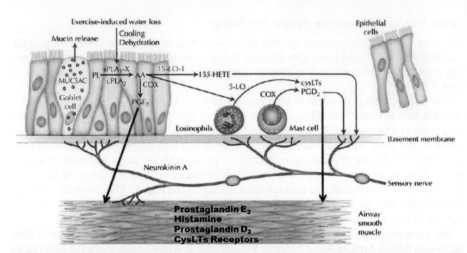

Fig. 2. Cells involved in exercise-induced bronchoconstriction. The epithelial cell layer is the source of prostaglandin E_2, a bronchodilating prostaglandin. The levels are lower in asthmatics. The mast cells are the source of prostaglandin D_2 and cysteinyl leukotrienes and eosinophils are also a source of cysteinyl leukotrienes. These bronchoconstricting mediators likely act via sensory nerves to cause smooth muscle contraction and airway narrowing. This phenomenon has been demonstrated indirectly by the increase in leukotrienes being related to the increase in mucin (MUC5A) released from goblet cells and the release of neurokinin A. The bronchial smooth muscle may also be stimulated directly by some of these same mediators. 5-LO, 5-lipoxygenase; COX, cyclooxygenase; PGD_2, prostaglandin D_2; PGE_2, prostaglandin E_2; PL, phospholipase; $sPLA_2$-X, secreted phospholipase A_2. (*From* Rundell KW, Anderson SD, Sue-Chu M, et al. Air quality and temperature effects on exercise-induced bronchoconstriction. Compr Physiol 2015;5(2):585; with permission.)

Temperature as a Modulator of Time Course and Severity of Exercise-Induced Bronchoconstriction

The severity of EIB is similar in the same individual over a wide range of inspired air temperatures, from cool (9°C) to hot (36°C; **Fig. 3**), providing that the inspired water content is low and remains the same.[7–9] This finding is consistent with the relatively constant value measured for water content of expired air (29–33 mg/L), when breathing air at 22°C to 40°C that contains less than 13 mg H_2O/L.[24] The maximum airway response is thought to occur when generations 10 to 12 are recruited, and this may take 8 minutes when the inspired air is warm. It is here, in the noncartilaginous airways, that the density of mast cells is high in individuals with asthma.[33] This finding may explain why warm dry air can still cause a similar decrease in expiratory flow to cool air.[8] The cooler the inspired air, the faster the required generations are recruited, and the earlier the response occurs.

EPITHELIAL DYSFUNCTION IN EXERCISE-INDUCED BRONCHOCONSTRICTION

The airway epithelium is the first structural barrier to the inhaled environment in the airway mucosa. Under normal circumstances, the epithelium forms a highly regulated and tight barrier that limits penetration of inhaled allergens, pathogens, pollutants, and other toxic compounds into the internal lung environment. Exercise hyperpnea can cause acute disruption of the airway epithelium.[34–36] The shedding of epithelial cells into the airway lumen after exercise challenge has been shown in individuals with asthma with EIB.[37] A (partial) loss of physical integrity of the epithelial barrier is likely to disrupt airway

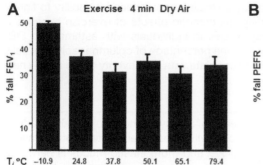

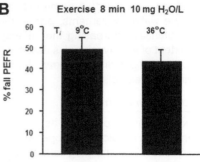

Fig. 3. The severity of the bronchoconstriction after exercise is similar in the same individual over a wide range of inspired air temperatures (T_i °C). (*A*) The reduction in forced expiratory volume in 1 second (FEV_1) after exercise expressed is a percentage of the preexercise level. (*B*) The reduction in peak expiratory flow rate (PEFR) is expressed as a percentage of the preexercise level. (*From [A]* Deal EC, McFadden ER, Ingram RH, et al. Role of respiratory heat exchange in production of exercise-induced asthma. J Appl Physiol Respir Environ Exerc Physiol 1979;46(3):467–75, with permission; and *From* Hahn A, Anderson SD, Morton AR, et al. A reinterpretation of the effect of temperature and water content of the inspired air in exercise-induced asthma. Am Rev Respir Dis 1984;130(4):575–9; Reprinted with permission of the American Thoracic Society. Copyright © 2018 American Thoracic Society. The American Journal of Respiratory and Critical Care Medicine is an official journal of the American Thoracic Society.)

homeostasis at a number of levels. Disruption of the ASL balance (resulting in malfunction of the mucociliary escalator), plasma exudation (resulting in edema), and attraction and activation of inflammatory cells in response to injury can all compromise airway homeostasis. Intrinsic dysfunction of the airway epithelium, as found in individuals with asthma,[38] and/or extreme levels of ventilation, as developed by endurance athletes,[39] are likely to increase the susceptibility to/extent of airway epithelial injury and, thereby, explain the high prevalence of EIB reported in both of these populations.[40,41]

Breaking Through the Epithelial Barrier

As minute ventilation increases during exercise, so does the load of foreign substances entering the airways. Disruption of epithelial tight junctions and/or gaps into the epithelium facilitates the penetration of foreign substances, enhancing the potential for toxic, immune, and inflammatory responses, with ensuing bronchoconstriction in susceptible individuals. During the pollen season, the severity of airway narrowing after outdoor exercise is increased in individuals with asthma with birch pollen allergy.[42] The cellular infiltration and activation of mast cells and T cells (and possibly eosinophils) observed during natural allergen exposure in atopic individuals with asthma[43] would render the airway smooth muscle more responsive to the stress of exercise. Further, common air pollutants and irritants (such as ozone or chlorine derivatives) have the potential per se to acutely disrupt the lung epithelial barrier.[44,45] Inhalation of noxious airborne agents during exercise hyperpnea could, therefore, aggravate the damage to the epithelium, and increase the risk/severity of EIB. In support of this concept, a high prevalence of EIB has consistently been reported in athletes who train and compete in polluted environments.[1]

Disturbance of the Airway Surface Liquid

Apart from being a barrier, the airway epithelium plays other roles, including maintenance of ASL levels.[46] Intact epithelial cells sense and autoregulate ASL height by active ion transport.[47] A damaged airway epithelium would loose its ability to tightly regulate water movements, potentiating the osmotic effects of exercise hyperpnea and potentially increasing the severity of EIB. In individuals with asthma with EIB, the extent of airway injury (as assessed by the percentage of columnar epithelial cells in sputum) at baseline has been shown to correlate with the severity of the airway narrowing after exercise.[29]

Mucus Dysfunction

Abnormal water movement, as a consequence of airway epithelial injury, also leads to alterations in rheological properties of mucus, with subsequent impairment of mucociliary clearance and plug formation. A thicker and more elastic mucus is harder to clear from the airways and provides an environment for microbial growth, leading to infection and inflammation.[48] In children with asthma (a population prone to EIB), viral infections of the airways are frequent and commonly associated with disease exacerbations.[49] Further, in elite athletes with asthma and/or EIB, an increase respiratory infection susceptibility has recently been reported.[50]

Mucus plugs could also contribute directly to lumenal obstruction in EIB. In individuals with asthma with EIB, exercise was found to initiate the release of MUC5AC (ie, the predominant gel-forming mucin of goblet cells).[51] Moreover, an hyperactivity of the mucus-secreting goblets has been reported in both individuals with asthma with EIB[51] and elite athletes.[52] Therefore, alterations in mucosal rheology secondary to epithelial dysfunction are likely to contribute to airflow obstruction and postexercise symptoms (such as cough and mucus hypersecretion).

Epithelial Damage Restitution

Restitution of the epithelium upon injury is associated with many tissue responses, including plasma exudation.[53] Plasma exudate in the airway lumen could not only contribute to EIB through mucosal/submucosal edema, but may also exacerbate some of the events described previously (ie, shedding of epithelium, impairment of mucociliary transport, and mucus plug formation).[54] Further, plasma exudate may cause airway inflammation and constriction owing to its content of powerful mediators.[53] In the context of elite sport, repeated plasma exudation has been proposed, via release of a wide range of chemoattractant factors and plasma proteins (such as cytokines and growth factors), to contribute to the development of EIB.[55] In elite athletes, late onset (>25 y) of EIB is common[56] and a change of the contractile properties of the airway smooth muscle is likely to result from combined effects of inflammatory and physical environmental stimuli. In asthma, owing to preexisting inflamed airways, the potent plasma-derived proteins–peptides released in response to hyperpnea-induced epithelial injury could activate an inflammatory cascade, with ensuing bronchoconstriction.

LEUKOCYTE ACTIVATION AS A FUNDAMENTAL MECHANISM OF EXERCISE-INDUCED BRONCHOCONSTRICTION
The Acute Response

There is strong evidence that the sustained bronchoconstriction after exercise and dry air hyperpnea challenges is due to the release of leukocyte-derived inflammatory mediators in the airways. Similar evidence indicates that hyperosmolar aerosols lead to the release of leukocyte-derived mediators.[28] Specifically, leukocyte-derived eicosanoids including the leukotrienes (LT) and prostaglandins (PG) play a pivotal role. After exercise challenge in asthmatics with EIB, there is sustained release of cysteinyl LTs (Cys-LTs, LTs C_4, D_4, and E_4) and PGD_2 into the conducting airways, corresponding with the development of acute bronchoconstriction.[29,31,57] The release of these mediators is attenuated under conditions that reduce the severity of EIB.[29,31,57,58] Pharmacologic inhibitors of this pathway unequivocally demonstrate that the release of these mediators play a causative role in the pathogenesis of EIB.[29,31,59] Inhibition of the key initial enzyme in LT biosynthesis, 5-lipoxygenase (5-LO) with either a 5-LO inhibitor or through inhibition of the 5-LO activating protein,[60] significantly reduces the severity of EIB.[61] Because LT receptor antagonists that block the Cys-LT$_1$ receptor similarly reduce the severity of EIB,[29,61] LTD$_4$ is likely to mediate bronchoconstriction (because LTD$_4$ is the primary agonist for the CysLT$_1$ receptor). However, the inhibition of EIB by LT modifiers is incomplete, implicating other bronchoconstrictive eicosanoids (such as PGD$_2$ and 15S-hydroxyeicosatetranoic acid [15S-HETE]), and/or the reduction in bronchoprotective mediators (such as PGE$_2$). PGD$_2$ binds to 2 major receptors, namely, DP1 and DP2, or CRTH2. There has been intense interest in development of CRTH2 inhibitors in chronic asthma because this receptor serves as a key regulator of leukocyte activation, but the results of such inhibitors for treatment of stable asthma have been modest.[62] With respect to EIB, the DP1 receptor may serve as the key receptor mediating bronchoconstriction and cough, because the DP1 receptor serves as a key activator of capsaicin sensitive sensory neurons (described elsewhere in this article).[63]

Although mediators that initiate bronchoconstriction directly are largely attributed to products derived by leukocytes, the epithelium can directly release mediators, such as 15S-HETE, and can serve as a source of the initial products of eicosanoid metabolism, leading to leukocyte-derived mediators by transcellular metabolism. In some cases, these alterations in eicosanoid synthesis can lead to shunting of arachidonic acid away from the production of PGE$_2$ and to an imbalance between the proinflammatory mediators, such as Cys-LTs relative to PGE$_2$.[64] In addition to the shunting of arachidonic acid away from PGE$_2$ production, there are other alterations in the epithelium under the influence of interleukin-13 that reduce the production of PGE$_2$.[65]

Mast cells and eosinophils are strongly implicated as the cellular sources of Cys-LTs and other eicosanoids (such as PGD$_2$) in EIB. After exercise challenge, histamine and the mast cell protease tryptase are released into the airways, demonstrating mast cell degranulation.[29] The eosinophil product eosinophilic cationic protein is released into the airways after a challenge, and the amount of eosinophilic cationic protein release varies with the severity of the EIB under different experimental conditions.[57] In analogous situations, pharmacologic inhibitors administered before mannitol and dry air hyperpnoea challenges revealed that histamine and possibly PGD$_2$ are responsible for the early onset of bronchoconstriction,[30,31,59] whereas the release of CysLTs is responsible for sustained bronchoconstriction.[30,66]

The Cellular and Molecular Phenotype Associated with Exercise-Induced Bronchoconstriction

The susceptibility to develop bronchoconstriction in response to hyperpnea challenge varies widely among subjects with established asthma and among individuals without a prior diagnosis of asthma. Thus, the presence of EIB after a specific challenge test represents a clinically recognizable phenotype of asthma. Recent work to understand the biological basis of this syndrome has revealed a consistent biological endotype related to cellular inflammation, particularly the density of mast cells in the airway epithelium.[67,68] Quantitative morphometry of airway biopsies, using design-based stereology, showed that the density of mast cells localized to the airway epithelium is significantly greater in subjects with EIB relative to individuals without asthma and those with asthma who do not have EIB (**Fig. 4**A, B).[69] Genome-wide expression studies of airway epithelial samples have also revealed high expression of the mast cell genes tryptase and

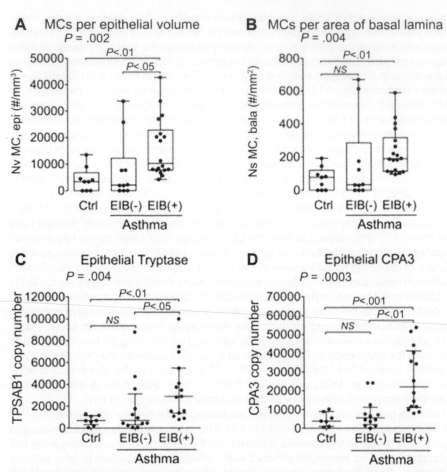

Fig. 4. Mast cell (MC) infiltration of the airway epithelium in asthma. Quantitative morphometry of endobronchial biopsy samples and epithelial brush gene expression from individuals without asthma (control [Ctrl]) compared with individuals with asthma and exercise-induced bronchoconstriction (EIB+) and individuals with asthma without EIB (EIB-). Quantitative morphometry reveals that (*A*) the number of mast cells per volume of airway epithelium and (*B*) the number of mast cells per area of the basal lamina (bala) are substantially increased in individuals with EIB compared with asthmatics without EIB and normal controls. Epithelial brushings show a pattern of mast cell gene expression of (*C*) tryptase and (*D*) carboxypeptidase A3 (CPA3) with high expression of these genes in EIB, but lower expression of chymase (data not shown). (*Adapted from* Lai Y, Altemeier WA, Vandree J, et al. Increased density of intraepithelial mast cells in exercise-induced bronchoconstriction regulated via epithelially-derived TSLP and IL-33. J Allergy Clin Immunol 2014;133(5):1451; with permission.)

carboxypeptidase A3, but low expression of chymase (**Fig. 4C, D**).[69,70] This unique intraepithelial mast cell phenotype is also a biomarker of the "Th2 high" molecular phenotype of asthma,[71,72] that is interleukin-13 mediated.[73,74] The association between airway eosinophilia and the severity of EIB also provides evidence of this association with "type 2" inflammation.[37,75] Further, modifications of airway proteins that reflect eosinophil activation are associated with the severity of EIB.[76] Individuals with EIB have higher levels of Cys-LTs in induced sputum[37] and in exhaled breath condensate.[77] Higher levels of Cys-LTs in this group likely reflects the ability of mast cells and eosinophils to direct the eicosanoid pathway toward the synthesis of Cys-LTs, because these cells are the predominant source of LTC_4 synthase, the key enzyme directing this pathway toward Cys-LT formation in the airways.[78] The rate-limiting step in eicosanoid formation occurs at the initial release of arachidonic acid by the hydrolysis of the sn-2 position of membrane phospholipids by a family of phospholipase A_2 (PLA_2) enzymes. Although the cytosolic PLA_2s (cPLA2) are known to serve this regulatory function, recent work has revealed that secreted PLA_2 ($sPLA_2$) activity is increased in asthma and is predominantly derived from $sPLA_2$ groups IIA and X (ie, $sPLA_2$-IIA and $sPLA_2$-X).[64,79] Further work has revealed that the level of $sPLA_2$-X is increased in the airways of subjects with asthma, and tends to be higher in subjects with EIB (**Fig. 5**).[80] In addition, $sPLA_2$-X is posttranslationally activated by transglutaminase 2, an enzyme that is overexpressed in the airways of patients with EIB.[70] Because the key source of $sPLA_2$-X is the epithelium, and the enzyme can serve as an activator of myeloid cells, such as eosinophils, to generate the production of Cys-LTs[81]; these results raise the possibility that $sPLA_2$-X serves as a critical initiator of eicosanoid production in response to exercise-induced hyperpnea.

Other markers of airway inflammation have also been associated with EIB, including an increase in the fraction of exhaled nitric oxide,[82] especially in subjects with atopy.[83] The levels of 8-isoprostanes, nonenzymatic products of phospholipid oxidation, are increased in the exhaled breath condensate of asthmatics with EIB, and correlated

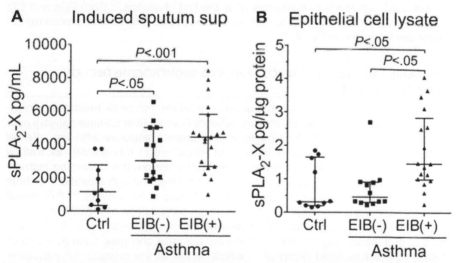

Fig. 5. Secreted phospholipase A_2 ($sPLA_2$-X) protein levels in the airways in asthma. Quantitative assessment of $sPLA_2$-X protein levels in induced sputum supernatant and lysates of epithelial brushings from the lower airways in individuals without asthma (control [Ctrl]) compared with individuals with asthma and exercise-induced bronchospasm (EIB+) and individuals with asthma without EIB (EIB-). (A) Induced sputum levels of $sPLA_2$-X were elevated in asthma, particularly in individuals with EIB. (B) The levels of $sPLA_2$-X in the epithelium were elevated only in the asthma group with EIB. (*Adapted from* Hallstrand TS, Lai Y, Altemeier WA, et al. Regulation and function of epithelial secreted phospholipase A2 group X in asthma. Am J Respir Crit Care Med 2013;188(1):45; Reprinted with permission of the American Thoracic Society. Copyright © 2018 American Thoracic Society. The American Journal of Respiratory and Critical Care Medicine is an official journal of the American Thoracic Society.)

with the severity of EIB.[84] A reduction in the level of the protective eicosanoid lipoxin A4 has also been described in EIB.[85]

In summary, patients who are susceptible to EIB have epithelial shedding, overproduction of inflammatory mediators such as Cys-LTs, relative underproduction of protective lipid mediators, and infiltration of the airways with eosinophils and mast cells (see **Fig. 2**).

Refractoriness to Repeated Exercise

A refractory period after EIB for approximately 2 hours occurs in 50% to 60% of people with asthma. This refractoriness is not due to a reduction in heat or water loss from the airways with repeated exercise. Many theories have been suggested to explain refractoriness.[86] The most compelling involve the release of mediators during exercise and their sustained presence after exercise. One theory relates to the bronchodilator effect of PGE_2 and the second relates to development of tolerance to the mediators of bronchoconstriction, particularly to the cysteinyl LTs. The finding that the nonsteroidal antiinflammatory agent indomethacin could prevent refractoriness to EIB was explained on the basis of blocking production of PGE_2 during initial challenge.[87] It is also known that refractoriness to exercise occurs after challenge with LTD_4.[88] Increased levels of PGE_2 have recently been reported during the refractory period after hyperpnea of dry air.[89] It has been proposed that repeated stimulation of the cysteinyl LT receptors lead to their internalization on the bronchial smooth muscle and would explain the refractoriness. When mediators were measured in response to repeated challenge with inhaled mannitol, the subjects most refractory to the second challenge had sustained high levels of mediators after the first challenge.[90] Both PGs and LTs work through G-protein–coupled receptors and the events proposed to explain refractoriness are illustrated in **Fig. 6**.[86]

NEUROGENIC FACTORS AND EXERCISE-INDUCED BRONCHOCONSTRICTION
Sensory Nerve Activation

The airways are innervated by network of sensory nerves that sense mechanical, nociceptive, and inflammatory signals through afferent C and A fibers. These sensory neurons send signals centrally, leading to a coordinated response with the efferent parasympathetic nervous system (described elsewhere in this article), as well as through a local reflex called retrograde axonal transmission. It is becoming increasingly clear that airway hyperresponsiveness is mediated through alterations in both the sensory and autonomic nervous system pathways in the airways.[91] This neural plasticity in asthma is the result of changes in the composition of the different types of sensory neurons, the production of neurokinins, such as neurokinin A and substance P, and the density of transient receptor potential channels, such as transient receptor potential vanilloid receptor 1, which serves as the receptor for capsaicin. These changes are the consequence of chronic inflammation and the generation of neurotropins, such as nerve growth factor.[92] In murine models, the sensory neurons are required for the development of airway hyperresponsiveness.[93] The precise anatomic changes in the sensory nervous system of the airways in human asthma are not known in detail; however, the threshold for activation of the sensory nerves by the transient receptor potential vanilloid receptor 1 agonist capsaicin is lowered in asthma.[94]

In animal models of EIB, it is well-established that the sensory nerves mediate bronchoconstriction in response to a period of dry air hyperpnea, and that the generation of leukocyte-derived eicosanoids plays the dominant role in activating this neural

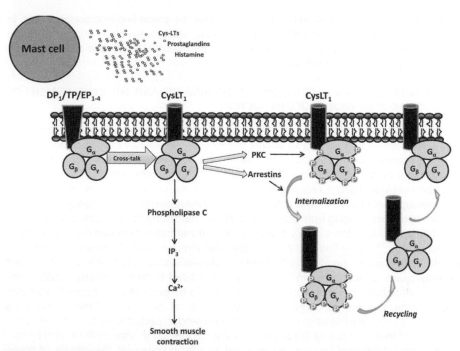

Fig. 6. Desensitization of Cys-LT1 as a mechanism of refractoriness. With exercise, there is release of cysteinyl leukotrienes from mast cells that stimulate the GPCR Cys-LT1 causing contraction of the muscle and exercise-induced bronchoconstriction. The prostaglandins generated during the same exercise could, via stimulation of the GPCRs DP1/EP1-4/TP, lead to cross-talk so that the Cys-LT1 is desensitized through phosphorylation and internalization. Refractoriness to a second exercise challenge within a short period occurs as a result. When the levels of mediators return to baseline values, the Cys-LT1 receptors are recycled back to the cell surface and the muscle becomes sensitive to further stimulation. When generation of prostaglandins is inhibited by agents, such as indomethacin and flurbiprofen, then there is limited desensitization of the Cys-LT1 and, therefore, limited refractoriness. Cys-LT$_1$, cysteinyl leukotriene receptor 1; DP$_1$, prostaglandin D receptor 1; EP$_{1-4}$, prostaglandin E receptor 1-4; GPCR, G-protein–coupled receptor; TP, thromboxane receptor. (*From* Larsson J, Anderson SD, Dahlén S-E, et al. Refractoriness to exercise challenge: a review of the mechanisms old and new. Immunol Allergy Clin N Am 2013;33(3):339; with permission.)

pathway. In a guinea pig model of hyperpnea-induced bronchoconstriction (HIB), inhibition of Cys-LT signaling, with either a 5-LO inhibitor or an LT receptor antagonist, inhibited HIB and the release of neurokinins, whereas a neurokinin 2 receptor antagonist inhibited HIB, but not the release of LTs, suggesting that LTs cause bronchoconstriction via sensory nerves during HIB.[95] In a dog model, a combination neurokinin 1 and 2 receptor antagonists inhibited HIB and the generation of LTs that are known in this model to cause HIB.[96] Sensory nerves are activated directly by osmotic stimuli, but several eicosanoids can either directly activate or alter the activation threshold of sensory nerves.[97] A recent study demonstrated that PGD$_2$, which is predominantly derived from mast cells, initiates sensory nerve activation through the DP1 receptor, regulating airway tone.[63] Although the function of neurokinins during EIB has not been tested fully, there is evidence that the levels of neurokinin A and Cys-LTs in the airways are correlated with the amount of bronchoconstriction after an exercise challenge and with the release of MUC5AC.[51] Overall, these findings suggest that, in humans, bronchoconstriction and mucus release after an exercise challenge is the consequence of sensory nerve activation that is initiated by the release of eicosanoids from airway leukocytes, such as mast cells.

THE ROLE OF REGIONAL ALTERATIONS IN THE AIRWAYS AND THE DEVELOPMENT OF EXERCISE-INDUCED BRONCHOCONSTRICTION

In model systems, particularly in animal models with either airway injury or inflamed airways, the mechanism leading to airway hyperresponsiveness includes regional alterations in airway diameter that are heterogenous, leading to the regional airway closure that contributes to the development of airflow obstruction.[98,99] With the use of hyperpolarized helium imaging to assess regional ventilation, it is apparent that the development of airflow obstruction after exercise represents heterogeneous effects on airway caliber, ranging from conducting airway narrowing to frank airway closure.[100] Treatment to reduce the severity of EIB reduces these heterogeneous regional defects in ventilation.[101] These findings suggest that the stimulus for EIB causes bronchoconstriction in regions of the airways that are specifically susceptible to this stimulus, most likely because of alterations in the airway wall related to airway inflammation. Such regional alterations in ventilation are also known to be present at baseline in subjects with asthma, and are associated with the severity of asthma.[102] There is evidence that areas of regional heterogeneity in ventilation tend to persist over time, further suggesting that these regions of the airways have a heightened susceptibility to airway narrowing.[103,32] Additional studies are needed to fully understand the nature of these regional alterations in airway structure and airway dysfunction in humans.

SUMMARY AND FUTURE CONSIDERATIONS

Water evaporation from the airways and thermal changes during exercise hyperpnea are well-established stimuli to EIB. In recent years, it has become increasingly clear that a dysfunctional airway epithelium, characterized by a loss of physical barrier integrity and impairment in signaling and secretory functions, renders individuals with asthma and elite athletes susceptible to EIB. In these 2 populations, lipid mediator release (cys-LTs and PGD$_2$) has repeatedly been observed in response to exercise challenge (or its surrogates), highlighting the inflammatory nature of the condition. Additional work is warranted to define the exact role of sensory nerves and of regional alterations in ventilation in the pathogenesis of EIB. Because EIB represents a precise asthma phenotype that can be characterized clinically, and is associated with an increasingly well-defined biological endotype, these findings should prove useful to target therapy for this important aspect of asthma.

REFERENCES

1. Rundell KW, Anderson SD, Sue-Chu M, et al. Air quality and temperature effects on exercise-induced bronchoconstriction. Compr Physiol 2015;5:579–610.
2. Deal EC, McFadden ER, Ingram RH, et al. Role of respiratory heat exchange in production of exercise-induced asthma. J Appl Physiol Respir Environ Exerc Physiol 1979;46:467–75.
3. McFadden ER, Lenner KA, Strohl KP. Postexertional airway rewarming and thermally induced asthma. J Clin Invest 1986;78(1):18–25.
4. McFadden ER, Gilbert IA. Exercise-induced asthma as a vascular phenomenon. Exercise-Induced Asthma 1999;130:115–35.

5. Gilbert IA, Fouke JM, McFadden ER. Heat and water flux in the intrathoracic airways and exercise-induced asthma. J Appl Physiol 1987;63(4):1681–91.
6. Anderson SD, Holzer K. Exercise-induced asthma: is it the right diagnosis in elite athletes? J Allergy Clin Immunol 2000;106(3):419–28.
7. Anderson SD, Schoeffel RE, Black JL, et al. Airway cooling as the stimulus to exercise-induced asthma - a re-evaluation. Eur J Respir Dis 1985;67(1):20–30.
8. Hahn A, Anderson SD, Morton AR, et al. A re-interpretation of the effect of temperature and water content of the inspired air in exercise-induced asthma. Am Rev Respir Dis 1984;130(4):575–9.
9. Eschenbacher WL, Moore TB, Lorenzen TJ, et al. Pulmonary responses of asthmatic and normal subjects to different temperature and humidity conditions in an environmental chamber. Lung 1992;170(1):51–62.
10. Zawadski DK, Lenner KA, McFadden ER. Comparison of intraairway temperatures in normal and asthmatic subjects after hyperpnea with hot, cold, and ambient air. Am Rev Respir Dis 1988;138(6):1553–8.
11. Strauss RH, McFadden ER, Ingram RH, et al. Influence of heat and humidity on the airway obstruction induced by exercise in asthma. J Clin Invest 1978;61(2):433–40.
12. Anderson SD, Schoeffel RE, Follet R, et al. Sensitivity to heat and water loss at rest and during exercise in asthmatic patients. Eur J Respir Dis 1982;63(5):459–71.
13. Anderson SD, Daviskas E, Schoeffel RE, et al. Prevention of severe exercise-induced asthma with hot humid air. Lancet 1979;2(8143):629.
14. Anderson SD. Is there a unifying hypothesis for exercise-induced asthma? J Allergy Clin Immunol 1984;73(5 Part 2):660–5.
15. Anderson SD, Daviskas E, Smith CM. Exercise-induced asthma: a difference in opinion regarding the stimulus. Allergy Proc 1989;10(3):215–26.
16. Anderson SD, Daviskas E. Pathophysiology of exercise-induced asthma: role of respiratory water loss. In: Weiler J, editor. Allergic and respiratory disease in sports medicine. New York: Marcel Dekker; 1997. p. 87–114.
17. McFadden ER Jr, Pichurko BM, Bowman HF, et al. Thermal mapping of the airways in humans. J Appl Physiol 1985;58(2):564–70.
18. Daviskas E, Gonda I, Anderson SD. Local airway heat and water vapour losses. Respir Physiol 1991;84(1):115–32.
19. Daviskas E, Gonda I, Anderson SD. Mathematical modelling of the heat and water transport in the human respiratory tract. J Appl Physiol 1990;69(1):362–72.
20. Davis MS, Daviskas E, Anderson SD, et al. Airway surface fluid desiccation during isocapnic hyperpnea. J Appl Physiol 2003;94(6):2545–7.
21. Daviskas E, Anderson SD, Gonda I, et al. Changes in mucociliary clearance during and after isocapnic hyperventilation in asthmatic and healthy subjects. Eur Respir J 1995;8(5):742–51.
22. Anderson SD, Daviskas E. The mechanism of exercise-induced asthma is .... J Allergy Clin Immunol 2000;106(3):453–9.
23. Anderson SD, Daviskas E. The airway microvasculature and exercise-induced asthma. Thorax 1992;47(9):748–52.
24. Anderson SD, Daviskas E. Airway drying and exercise induced asthma. In: McFadden ER, editor. Exercise induced asthma - lung biology in health and disease. New York: Marcel Dekker; 1999. p. 77–113.
25. Agostoni P, Arena V, Doria E, et al. Inspired gas relative humidity affects systemic to pulmonary bronchial blood flow in humans. Chest 1990;97(6):1377–80.

26. Smith CM, Anderson SD. A comparison between the airway response to iso-capnic hyperventilation and hypertonic saline in subjects with asthma. Eur Respir J 1989;2(1):36–43.

27. Gibson PG, Saltos N, Borgas T. Airway mast cells and eosinophils correlate with clinical severity and airway hyperresponsiveness in corticosteroid-treated asthma. J Allergy Clin Immunol 2000;105(4):752–9.

28. Brannan JD, Gulliksson M, Anderson SD, et al. Evidence of mast cell activation and leukotriene release after mannitol inhalation. Eur Respir J 2003;22(3): 491–6.

29. Hallstrand TS, Moody MW, Wurfel MM, et al. Inflammatory basis of exercise-induced bronchoconstriction. Am J Respir Crit Care Med 2005;172(6):679–86.

30. Brannan JD, Gulliksson M, Anderson SD, et al. Inhibition of mast cell PGD_2 release protects against mannitol-induced airway narrowing. Eur Respir J 2006;27(5):944–50.

31. Kippelen P, Larsson J, Anderson SD, et al. Effect of sodium cromoglycate on mast cell mediators during hyperpnea in athletes. Med Sci Sports Exerc 2010;42(10):1853–60.

32. Hallstrand TS. New insights into pathogenesis of exercise-induced bronchocon-striction. Curr Opin Allergy Clin Immunol 2012;12(1):42–8.

33. Carroll NG, Mutavdzic S, James AL. Distribution and degranulation of airway mast cells in normal and asthmatic subjects. Eur Respir J 2002;19(5):879–85.

34. Chimenti L, Morici G, Paternò A, et al. Bronchial epithelial damage after a half-marathon in nonasthmatic amateur runners. Am J Physiol Lung Cell Mol Physiol 2010;298(6):L857–62.

35. Bolger C, Tufvesson E, Sue-Chu M, et al. Hyperpnea-induced bronchoconstric-tion and urinary CC16 levels in athletes. Med Sci Sports Exerc 2011;43(7): 1207–13.

36. Bolger C, Tufvesson E, Anderson SD, et al. Effect of inspired air conditions on exercise-induced bronchoconstriction and urinary CC16 levels in athletes. J Appl Physiol (1985) 2011;111(4):1059–65.

37. Hallstrand TS, Moody MW, Aitken ML, et al. Airway immunopathology of asthma with exercise-induced bronchoconstriction. J Allergy Clin Immunol 2005;116(3): 586–93.

38. Holgate ST. Epithelium dysfunction in asthma. J Allergy Clin Immunol 2007; 120(6):1233–44 [quiz: 45–6].

39. Anderson SD, Kippelen P. Airway injury as a mechanism for exercise-induced bronchoconstriction in elite athletes. J Allergy Clin Immunol 2008;122(2): 225–35 [quiz: 36–7].

40. Carlsen KH, Anderson SD, Bjermer L, et al. Exercise-induced asthma, respira-tory and allergic disorders in elite athletes: epidemiology, mechanisms and diagnosis: part I of the report from the joint task force of the European Respira-tory Society (ERS) and the European Academy of Allergy and Clinical Immu-nology (EAACI) in cooperation with GA2LEN. Allergy 2008;63(4):387–403.

41. Cabral AL, Conceição GM, Fonseca-Guedes CH, et al. Exercise-induced bron-chospasm in children: effects of asthma severity. Am J Respir Crit Care Med 1999;159(6):1819–23.

42. Karjalainen J, Lindqvist A, Laitinen LA. Seasonal variability of exercise-induced asthma especially outdoors. Effect of birch pollen allergy. Clin Exp Allergy 1989; 19(3):273–8.

43. Djukanović R, Feather I, Gratziou C, et al. Effect of natural allergen exposure during the grass pollen season on airways inflammatory cells and asthma symptoms. Thorax 1996;51(6):575–81.
44. Carbonnelle S, Francaux M, Doyle I, et al. Changes in serum pneumoproteins caused by short-term exposures to nitrogen trichloride in indoor chlorinated swimming pools. Biomarkers 2002;7(6):464–78.
45. Krishna MT, Springall D, Meng QH, et al. Effects of ozone on epithelium and sensory nerves in the bronchial mucosa of healthy humans. Am J Respir Crit Care Med 1997;156(3 Pt 1):943–50.
46. Matsui H, Davis CW, Tarran R, et al. Osmotic water permeabilities of cultured, well-differentiated normal and cystic fibrosis airway epithelia. J Clin Invest 2000;105(10):1419–27.
47. Tarran R. Regulation of airway surface liquid volume and mucus transport by active ion transport. Proc Am Thorac Soc 2004;1(1):42–6.
48. Fahy JV, Dickey BF. Airway mucus function and dysfunction. N Engl J Med 2010; 363(23):2233–47.
49. Olenec JP, Kim WK, Lee WM, et al. Weekly monitoring of children with asthma for infections and illness during common cold seasons. J Allergy Clin Immunol 2010;125(5):1001–6.e1.
50. Bonini M, Gramiccioni C, Fioretti D, et al. Asthma, allergy and the Olympics: a 12-year survey in elite athletes. Curr Opin Allergy Clin Immunol 2015;15(2): 184–92.
51. Hallstrand TS, Debley JS, Farin FM, et al. Role of MUC5AC in the pathogenesis of exercise-induced bronchoconstriction. J Allergy Clin Immunol 2007;119(5): 1092–8.
52. Bougault V, Loubaki L, Joubert P, et al. Airway remodeling and inflammation in competitive swimmers training in indoor chlorinated swimming pools. J Allergy Clin Immunol 2012;129(2):351–8.e1.
53. Persson CG, Erjefält JS, Andersson M, et al. Extravasation, lamina propria flooding and lumenal entry of bulk plasma exudate in mucosal defence, inflammation and repair. Pulm Pharmacol 1996;9(3):129–39.
54. Persson CG. Plasma exudation and asthma. Lung 1988;166(1):1–23.
55. Anderson SD, Kippelen P. Exercise-induced bronchoconstriction: pathogenesis. Curr Allergy Asthma Rep 2005;5(2):116–22.
56. Fitch KD. An overview of asthma and airway hyper-responsiveness in Olympic athletes. Br J Sports Med 2012;46(6):413–6.
57. Mickleborough TD, Lindley MR, Ray S. Dietary salt, airway inflammation, and diffusion capacity in exercise-induced asthma. Med Sci Sports Exerc 2005; 37(6):904–14.
58. Simpson AJ, Bood JR, Anderson SD, et al. A standard, single dose of inhaled terbutaline attenuates hyperpnea-induced bronchoconstriction and mast cell activation in athletes. J Appl Physiol (1985) 2016;120(9):1011–7.
59. Kippelen P, Larsson J, Anderson SD, et al. Acute effects of beclomethasone on hyperpnea-induced bronchoconstriction. Med Sci Sports Exerc 2010;42(2): 273–80.
60. Kent SE, Bentley JH, Miller D, et al. The effect of GSK2190915, a 5-lipoxygenase-activating protein inhibitor, on exercise-induced bronchoconstriction. Allergy Asthma Proc 2014;35(2):126–33.
61. Hallstrand TS, Henderson WR. Role of leukotrienes in exercise-induced bronchoconstriction. Curr Allergy Asthma Rep 2009;9(1):18–25.

62. Farne H, Jackson DJ, Johnston SL. Are emerging PGD2 antagonists a promising therapy class for treating asthma? Expert Opin Emerg Drugs 2016;21(4): 359–64.

63. Maher SA, Birrell MA, Adcock JJ, et al. Prostaglandin D2 and the role of the DP1, DP2 and TP receptors in the control of airway reflex events. Eur Respir J 2015;45(4):1108–18.

64. Hallstrand TS, Chi EY, Singer AG, et al. Secreted phospholipase A2 group X overexpression in asthma and bronchial hyperresponsiveness. Am J Respir Crit Care Med 2007;176(11):1072–8.

65. Trudeau J, Hu H, Chibana K, et al. Selective downregulation of prostaglandin E_2-related pathways by the Th2 cytokine IL-13. J Allergy Clin Immunol 2006;117(6): 1446–54.

66. Currie GP, Haggart K, Lee DK, et al. Effects of mediator antagonism on mannitol and adenosine monophosphate challenges. Clin Exp Allergy 2003;33(6):783–8.

67. Lötvall J, Akdis CA, Bacharier LB, et al. Asthma endotypes: a new approach to classification of disease entities within the asthma syndrome. J Allergy Clin Immunol 2011;127(2):355–60.

68. Wenzel SE. Asthma phenotypes: the evolution from clinical to molecular approaches. Nat Med 2012;18(5):716–25.

69. Lai Y, Altemeier WA, Vandree J, et al. Increased density of intraepithelial mast cells in patients with exercise-induced bronchoconstriction regulated through epithelially derived thymic stromal lymphopoietin and IL-33. J Allergy Clin Immunol 2014;133(5):1448–55.

70. Hallstrand TS, Wurfel MM, Lai Y, et al. Transglutaminase 2, a novel regulator of eicosanoid production in asthma revealed by genome-wide expression profiling of distinct asthma phenotypes. PLoS One 2010;5(1):e8583.

71. Dougherty RH, Sidhu SS, Raman K, et al. Accumulation of intraepithelial mast cells with a unique protease phenotype in T(H)2-high asthma. J Allergy Clin Immunol 2010;125(5):1046–53.e8.

72. Woodruff PG, Boushey HA, Dolganov GM, et al. Genome-wide profiling identifies epithelial cell genes associated with asthma and with treatment response to corticosteroids. Proc Natl Acad Sci U S A 2007;104(40):15858–63.

73. Woodruff PG, Modrek B, Choy DF, et al. T-helper type 2-driven inflammation defines major subphenotypes of asthma. Am J Respir Crit Care Med 2009;180(5): 388–95.

74. Peters MC, Mekonnen ZK, Yuan S, et al. Measures of gene expression in sputum cells can identify TH2-high and TH2-low subtypes of asthma. J Allergy Clin Immunol 2014;133(2):388–94.

75. Duong M, Subbarao P, Adelroth E, et al. Sputum eosinophils and the response of exercise-induced bronchoconstriction to corticosteroid in asthma. Chest 2008;133(2):404–11.

76. Jin H, Hallstrand TS, Daly DS, et al. A halotyrosine antibody that detects increased protein modifications in asthma patients. J Immunol Methods 2014; 403(1–2):17–25.

77. Carraro S, Corradi M, Zanconato S, et al. Exhaled breath condensate cysteinyl leukotrienes are increased in children with exercise-induced bronchoconstriction. J Allergy Clin Immunol 2005;115(4):764–70.

78. Cai Y, Bjermer L, Halstensen TS. Bronchial mast cells are the dominating LTC_4S-expressing cells in aspirin-tolerant asthma. Am J Respir Cell Mol Biol 2003; 29(6):683–93.

79. Hallstrand TS, Lai Y, Ni Z, et al. Relationship between levels of secreted phospholipase A groups IIA and X in the airways and asthma severity. Clin Exp Allergy 2011;41(6):801–10.

80. Hallstrand TS, Lai Y, Altemeier WA, et al. Regulation and function of epithelial secreted phospholipase A2 group X in asthma. Am J Respir Crit Care Med 2013;188(1):42–50.

81. Lai Y, Oslund RC, Bollinger JG, et al. Eosinophil cysteinyl leukotriene synthesis mediated by exogenous secreted phospholipase A2 group X. J Biol Chem 2010;285(53):41491–500.

82. Scollo M, Zanconato S, Ongaro R, et al. Exhaled nitric oxide and exercise-induced bronchoconstriction in asthmatic children. Am J Respir Crit Care Med 2000;161(3 Pt 1):1047–50.

83. Malmberg LP, Pelkonen AS, Mattila PS, et al. Exhaled nitric oxide and exercise-induced bronchoconstriction in young wheezy children - interactions with atopy. Pediatr Allergy Immunol 2009;20(7):673–8.

84. Barreto M, Villa MP, Olita C, et al. 8-Isoprostane in exhaled breath condensate and exercise-induced bronchoconstriction in asthmatic children and adolescents. Chest 2009;135(1):66–73.

85. Tahan F, Saraymen R, Gumus H. The role of lipoxin A4 in exercise-induced bronchoconstriction in asthma. J Asthma 2008;45(2):161–4.

86. Larsson J, Anderson SD, Dahlen SE, et al. Refractoriness to exercise challenge: a review of the mechanisms old and new. Immunol Allergy Clin N Am 2013;33: 329–45.

87. O'Byrne PM, Jones GL. The effect of indomethacin on exercise-induced bronchoconstriction and refractoriness after exercise. Am Rev Respir Dis 1986; 134(1):69–72.

88. Manning PJ, Watson RM, O'Byrne PM. Exercise-induced refractoriness in asthmatic subjects involves leukotriene and prostaglandin interdependent mechanisms. Am Rev Respir Dis 1993;148(4 Pt 1):950–4.

89. Bood JR, Sundblad BM, Delin I, et al. Urinary excretion of lipid mediators in response to repeated eucapnic voluntary hyperpnea in asthmatic subjects. J Appl Physiol (1985) 2015;119(3):272–9.

90. Larsson J, Perry CP, Anderson SD, et al. The occurrence of refractoriness and mast cell mediator release following mannitol-induced bronchoconstriction. J Appl Physiol 2011;110:1029–35.

91. Zaccone EJ, Undem BJ. Airway vagal neuroplasticity associated with respiratory viral infections. Lung 2016;194(1):25–9.

92. Ogawa H, Azuma M, Uehara H, et al. Nerve growth factor derived from bronchial epithelium after chronic mite antigen exposure contributes to airway hyperresponsiveness by inducing hyperinnervation, and is inhibited by in vivo siRNA. Clin Exp Allergy 2012;42(3):460–70.

93. Trankner D, Hahne N, Sugino K, et al. Population of sensory neurons essential for asthmatic hyperreactivity of inflamed airways. Proc Natl Acad Sci U S A 2014;111(31):11515–20.

94. Belvisi MG, Birrell MA, Khalid S, et al. Neurophenotypes in airway diseases. Insights from translational cough studies. Am J Respir Crit Care Med 2016; 193(12):1364–72.

95. Lai YL, Lee SP. Mediators in hyperpnea-induced bronchoconstriction of guinea pigs. Naunyn Schmiedebergs Arch Pharmacol 1999;360(5):597–602.

96. Freed AN, McCulloch S, Meyers T, et al. Neurokinins modulate hyperventilation-induced bronchoconstriction in canine peripheral airways. Am J Respir Crit Care Med 2003;167(8):1102–8.
97. Taylor-Clark TE, Nassenstein C, Undem BJ. Leukotriene D4 increases the excitability of capsaicin-sensitive nasal sensory nerves to electrical and chemical stimuli. Br J Pharmacol 2008;154(6):1359–68.
98. Lundblad LK, Thompson-Figueroa J, Allen GB, et al. Airway hyperresponsiveness in allergically inflamed mice: the role of airway closure. Am J Respir Crit Care Med 2007;175(8):768–74.
99. Bates JH, Cojocaru A, Haverkamp HC, et al. The synergistic interactions of allergic lung inflammation and intratracheal cationic protein. Am J Respir Crit Care Med 2008;177(3):261–8.
100. Samee S, Altes T, Powers P, et al. Imaging the lungs in asthmatic patients by using hyperpolarized helium-3 magnetic resonance: assessment of response to methacholine and exercise challenge. J Allergy Clin Immunol 2003;111(6):1205–11.
101. Kruger SJ, Niles DJ, Dardzinski B, et al. Hyperpolarized Helium-3 MRI of exercise-induced bronchoconstriction during challenge and therapy. J Magn Reson Imaging 2014;39(5):1230–7.
102. de Lange EE, Altes TA, Patrie JT, et al. Evaluation of asthma with hyperpolarized helium-3 MRI: correlation with clinical severity and spirometry. Chest 2006;130(4):1055–62.
103. Niles DJ, Kruger SJ, Dardzinski BJ, et al. Exercise-induced bronchoconstriction: reproducibility of hyperpolarized 3He MR imaging. Radiology 2013;266(2):618–25.

Exercise-Induced Bronchoconstriction and the Air We Breathe

Kenneth W. Rundell, PhD[a],*, James M. Smoliga, DVM, PhD[b],
Valérie Bougault, PhD[c]

KEYWORDS

- Air pollution • Particulate matter • Ozone • Trichloramines • Nitrogen dioxide
- Sulfur dioxide • Exercise-induced bronchoconstriction • Asthma

KEY POINTS

- Environmental factors that influence mediator release and airway pathology include ambient air humidity and airborne pollutants, including chemical irritants and particulate matter.
- The high ventilatory demands of exercise exacerbates total exposure to noxious stimuli and allows particulate matter to deposit at deeper levels within the lungs.
- Subjects with and without respiratory pathologies may present respiratory symptoms in polluted environments or cold, dry air.
- The prevalence of exercise-induced bronchoconstriction and asthma in competitive athletes is attributed to training and competing in adverse environmental conditions.
- New-onset asthma from chronic inhalation of pollutants and the acute exercise-induced bronchoconstriction response is a major health concern for individuals training, competing, working, and recreating in high pollution environments.

INTRODUCTION

Exercise-induced bronchoconstriction (EIB) is defined as the transient abnormal constriction of the airways in response to vigorous exercise.[1] Key mediators in this response are histamine, leukotrienes, and prostaglandins that are released from mast cells, eosinophils and neutrophils in the airways.[2,3] These mediators are released in response to the airway mucosa being exposed to various triggers related to air

Disclosure Statement: The authors have no conflicts of interest.
[a] Department of Basic Sciences, Geisinger Commonwealth School of Medicine, 525 Pine Street, Scranton, PA 18510, USA; [b] Department of Physical Therapy, High Point University, 1 University Parkway, High Point, NC 27262, USA; [c] Pluridisciplinary Research Unit Sport, University of Lille, Health Society (URePSSS), EA7369, Lille, France
* Corresponding author. 605 Skyline Drive South, South Abington Township, PA 18411.
E-mail address: kwrundell@gmail.com

Immunol Allergy Clin N Am 38 (2018) 183–204
https://doi.org/10.1016/j.iac.2018.01.009   immunology.theclinics.com

quality. Environmental factors that influence mediator release include ambient air humidity and airborne pollutants, including chemical irritants and particulate matter (PM).[4,5] The high ventilatory demands of exercise exacerbates total exposure to these noxious stimuli, while also allowing PM to deposit at deeper levels within the lungs.[6]

Although acute exposure to these environmental triggers is capable of initiating an EIB event, chronic exposure is epidemiologically linked to the development of asthma and other allergic/immunologic conditions. The prevalence of EIB and asthma in competitive athletes exceeds that found in the recreational athlete, and has been attributed to training and competing in adverse environmental conditions,[1] such as the high pollution conditions found in ice rinks, indoor swimming pools, and high vehicular traffic areas.[7] New-onset asthma from the chronic inhalation of pollutants and the acute EIB response present a major health concern for individuals training, competing, working, and recreating in these high pollutant environments. Thus, this paper aims to explore the relationship between EIB and asthma with specific environmental exposures commonly encountered during exercise, in the hopes that a greater understanding of these associations can lead to improved prevention and clinical management of airway disease.

GENERAL PATHOGENESIS OF POLLUTION-INDUCED AIRWAY DYSFUNCTION
Oxidative Stress

There is increasing evidence supporting the notion that oxidative stress caused by the inhalation of environmental pollutants during exercise promotes the development of asthma and enhances the EIB response.[8–12] Oxidative stress is a key feature in the pathogenesis of asthma[13] and is likely involved in the production and release of inflammatory mediators in the EIB response.[14] The oxidative stress in the airways includes the increase in reactive oxygen/nitrogen species (RONS) concomitant with a decrease in resident antioxidants. Increased concentrations of 8-isoprostane, a marker of airway oxidative stress, in exhaled breath condensate are associated with EIB.[14] Additionally, plasma and exhaled breath condensate concentrations of biomarkers associated with lipid peroxidation, such as malondialdehyde, are increased after exercise in athletes with EIB.[15]

Inflammation

The biologic response to the inhalation of air pollution has been shown to stimulate airway inflammation through oxidative stress and is characterized by an increase in airway inflammatory cells and inflammatory mediators (**Fig. 1**). Pollution exposure (fine particles, particles <2.5 μm and >0.1 μm in diameter, [$PM_{2.5}$], diesel exhaust, ozone) has been associated with increased neutrophils, eosinophils, eosinophil cationic protein, interleukin (IL)-8, and IL-33 in nasal lavage, in vitro animal studies, and human bronchial lavage samples.[16–19] Increases in myeloperoxidase, neutrophils, mast cells, CD4+ and CD8+ T lymphocytes, and the upregulation of adhesion molecules (eg, intercellular adhesion molecule-1 and vascular cell adhesion molecule-1) have been associated with ultrafine particle exposure,[20,21] supporting neutrophilic inflammation in the airways.[18,22,23]

Glutathione Depletion

Reduced glutathione (GSH) plays a central role in protection against airway oxidative stress and has been shown to decrease in asthmatics[24] and after PM exposure in airway epithelial cells in vitro.[25] Conversely, GSH may increase in healthy subjects after exposure to mild levels of diesel exhaust, indicating that the air–lung interface in

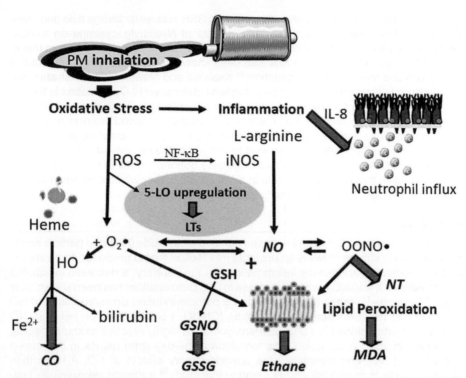

Fig. 1. Possible pathways from particulate matter (PM)-induced oxidative stress initiating airway inflammation, damage, and bronchoconstriction. GSH, glutathione; GSNO, nitroso-glutathione; GSSG, oxidized glutathione; IL-8, interleukin-8; iNOS, inducible nitric oxide; LTs, leukotrienes; MDA, malondialdehyde; NF-κB, nuclear factor κB; NO, nitric oxide; NT, nitrotyrosine; ROS, reactive oxygen species. (*Adapted from* Paredi P, Kharitonov SA, Barnes PJ. Analysis of expired air for oxidation products. Am J Respir Crit Care Med 2002;166(12 Pt 2):S32; Reprinted with permission of the American Thoracic Society. Copyright © 2018 American Thoracic Society. The American Journal of Respiratory and Critical Care Medicine is an official journal of the American Thoracic Society.)

healthy subjects is capable of counteracting an acute mild oxidative challenge.[26] Thus, GSH is a critical antioxidant in the airways. Decreased GSH has been shown in various lung dysfunctions, whereas oxidized GSH has been found to be high in the bronchial fluids of asthmatics.[24] It has been suggested that low GSH in the lung may amplify inflammation and airway hyperresponsiveness (AHR).[27] It seems likely that the airway dysfunction attributed to PM exposure is related to GSH status.

Antioxidant defense pathways[28] and GSH homeostasis[29] are controlled by GSH S-transferase, which is found in high concentrations in the lung. The single nucleotide polymorphism of GSH S-transferase π (GSTP1) ile^{105} has been linked to the development of new-onset asthma and EIB in children who participate in team sports in high ambient ozone, demonstrating a hazard ratio for new-onset asthma of 6.15 (95% confidence interval, 2.2–7.4).[30] Thus, genotypic variation can account for some of the interindividual variation in respiratory responses to pollution exposure.

Evidence supporting the clinical importance of airway GSH can be found in studies using the GSH precursor N-acetyl-L-cysteine. Treatment with the cysteine donor (in the synthesis of GSH) N-acetyl-L-cysteine has been used therapeutically to reduce inflammation in various lung diseases. Results have been promising; Meyer and colleagues[31] have shown a significant increase in GSH in alveolar lavage fluid and other studies[32–35] have demonstrated beneficial effects of N-acetyl-L-cysteine on oxidant mediated lung inflammation and inhibition of nuclear factor κB and IL-8 upregulation. The cysteine donor N-acystelyn has also been shown to increase lung epithelial cell GSH levels and inhibit RONS production.[34] Kasielski and Nowak[35] demonstrated that long-term oral administration of N-acetyl-cysteine attenuated H_2O_2 formation in the airways of patients with chronic obstructive pulmonary disease. Rubio and colleagues[36] demonstrated oral N-acetyl-cysteine attenuated elastase-induced pulmonary emphysema in rats. Blesa and associates[32] demonstrated that oral N-acetyl-cysteine attenuates pulmonary inflammation in response to antigen in the rat. Several in vitro studies have demonstrated similar effects by the cysteine donors.[37,38] All of these studies are suggestive of RONS having a key role in airway dysfunction, which can potentially be attenuated through therapeutics that support GSH function.

Nitric Oxide

Marginal associations between increased exhaled nitric oxide (NO) and particle exposure have been shown.[39] NO is an unstable free radical that is proposed to be important in vasodilation and airway inflammation. On the contrary, a decrease in exhaled NO, alveolar NO, and NO_3, with an increase in lipid peroxidation, has been shown after high PM exercise[15]; these findings support a particle-induced downregulation of NO synthase and the formation of peroxynitrite (ONOO−) by the reaction between NO and super oxide anions (O_2^-) (**Fig. 2**). Peroxynitrite, a highly reactive oxidant species, is involved in lipid peroxidation. The formation of peroxynitrite results in decreased availability of NO, and diminishes the provasodilatory effects of NO. A more than 200% increase in malondialdehyde found in this study[15] supports peroxynitrite initiated lipid peroxidation.[40] The significant correlations between lung function and change in NO_3 and exhaled NO in this study[15] support a mechanism of decreased NO availability causing a sympathetic-induced bronchoconstriction or vasoconstriction. That finding provides a plausible explanation for the reduction in carbon monoxide diffusing capacity and decreased mid expiratory flow rates after ultrafine particle inhalation noted by Pietropaoli and colleagues.[41]

Likewise, NO reacts with GSH to form a potent airway bronchodilator, S-nitrosoglutathione (GSNO).[42,43] It has been proposed that GSNO is critical in the AHR characteristic of asthma.[43] An in vitro study[44] using cultured alveolar macrophage cells demonstrated pronounced interaction between S-nitrosothiol metabolism and leukotriene metabolism. This study found that low levels of GSNO (0.5–1.0 μmol/L) increase 5-lipoxygenase expression, whereas levels exceeding 5 μmol/L inhibit 5-lipoxygenase expression and activity.[44] 5-Lipoxygenase is the rate-limiting enzyme in the biosynthesis of the potent bronchoconstrictors, cysteinyl leukotrienes. In support of this finding, Que and colleagues[43] demonstrated that endogenous GSNO (when not broken down by GSNO reductase) protects against methacholine-induced AHR and augments β2-andrenergic agonist airway relaxation. A decrease in GSNO may in part explain why leukotrienes are predominant mediators in PM-induced bronchoconstriction.[5]

EXPOSURE-SPECIFIC PATHOPHYSIOLOGY
Exercise-Induced Bronchospasm and Environmental Humidity and Temperature

Ambient air humidity is a key factor in the onset of bronchoconstriction. Generally speaking, this constriction occurs as a result of local changes in airway surface liquid osmolarity from conditioning large volumes of inspired air to body temperature and

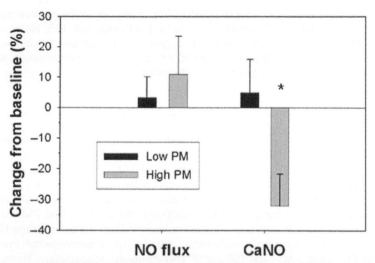

Fig. 2. The small decrease in exhaled nitric oxide (eNO) after high PM_1 (PM < 1 micrometer diameter) exercise was not different from the small decrease after low PM_1 exercise. Conducting airways nitric oxide (NO) flux was also not different between exposures, but fractional alveolar contribution to eNO (CaNO) significantly decreased 32% after high PM_1 exercise ($P = .02$). Exhaled NO was determined at 5 flow rates to calculate NO flux (nL s^{-1}) and CaNO (parts per billion). A plot of NO output (nL s^{-1}) versus expiratory flow rate (mL s^{-1}) was used to calculate NO flux and CaNO. The volume of eNO (VeNO) was calculated by multiplying the fraction of eNO plateau values by the expiratory flow rates. Linear least squares method was used to determine the best fit line through a plot of VeNO versus flow rate. NO flux was indicated as the y intercept and CaNO was indicated as the slope of the line. The decrease in eNO was attributed to CaNO, but not to conducting airway NO flux and the decrease in NO_3 and eNO combined with a large increase in malondialdehyde could provide a plausible pathway for peroxynitrite-mediated lipid peroxidation. * $P < .05$ (*From* Rundell KW, Slee JB, Caviston R, et al. Decreased lung function after inhalation of ultrafine and fine particulate matter during exercise is related to decreased total nitrate in exhaled breath condensate. Inhal Toxicol 2008;20(1):5; with permission.)

99% relative humidity during exercise.[45,46] The change in osmolarity causes resident inflammatory cells to degranulate, releasing inflammatory cell mediators that act on responsive bronchial smooth muscle receptors.[47] Cold air is generally associated with EIB, but this is generally due to the low water content of cold air rather than the temperature itself. Even if air is warmed to body temperature, an EIB response can be observed in asthmatics; however, the response is attenuated when the air is humidified.[48] Thus, endurance athletes training in cold environments (eg, cross-country skiers) are at increased risk of EIB, as well as the development of asthma.[49,50] Cross-country skiers without a history or EIB or asthma experience airway inflammation and remodeling similar to individuals with frank asthma.[51] Such macroscopic inflammatory changes have been observed in a cohort adolescent skiers (mean of 7 years of experience) compared with controls, and this inflammation was worse in skiers with asthma.[52] Airway remodeling and consequent signs and symptoms of pulmonary dysfunction in these athletes may occur in the presence[53] or absence of bronchial hypersensitivity.[54] This remodeling may result in progressive decreases in pulmonary function, as evidenced by an increased prevalence of self-reported asthma with age in skiers.[49] Additionally, Stensrud and coworkers[55] reported that exercise performance is decreased by approximately 5% in dry air (40% relative humidity) compared with humid air (95% relative humidity) in athletes with EIB. However, in a recent systemic review by Price and colleagues,[56] the authors concluded that, although it is reasonable to suspect that EIB impacts athletic performance, there is currently insufficient evidence to provide a definitive answer.

Particulate Matter

Airborne PM consists of a mixture of small particles of organic and inorganic compounds, acids, metal, dust, and carbon. PM is categorized as course particles (PM_{10}; 2.5–10 μm diameter), fine particles ($PM_{2.5}$), and nano/ultrafine size ($PM_{0.1}$; <0.1 μm diameter; **Fig. 3**). The primary source of $PM_{2.5}$ and ultrafine particles is from fossil fuel combustion emissions such as motor vehicles, furnaces, and gas cooking stoves. Greater than 90% of the particles from diesel emissions are in the ultrafine size range,[57] and current thinking supports the concept that PM toxicity is related to smaller particle size and number count.[20,58] The 24-hour average National Ambient Air Quality Standards established by the US Environmental Protection Agency for PM_{10} and $PM_{2.5}$ are 150 μg/m³ and 35 μg/m³, respectively. There are no standards for $PM_{0.1}$ because a mass metric for these does not provide practical information; these nano/ultrafine particles are best described by a number metric (particles/cm³). However, the small size and mass of these smallest particles allows them to have the greatest alveolar deposition, which is exacerbated by the high ventilations of exercise.[6,59] Daigle and colleagues[6] examined lung deposition of ultrafine carbon black particles (mean diameter, 26 ± 1.6 nm) at rest and during moderate exercise; the number of particles deposited during exercise was 4.5-fold greater than at rest and was attributed to the combined increase in deposition fraction during exercise (from 0.66 ± 0.11 to 0.83 ± 0.04) and increased minute ventilation during exercise (from 9.0 ± 1.3 to 38.1 ± 9.5 L/min). This may have implications to respiratory health of those exercising in areas of high airborne PM. PM generated from combustion emissions can be associated with the formation of RONS and influence mediators released from airway cells involved in EIB.[15,60,61] Exposure to PM has been associated with emergency department visits,[62,63] increased bronchodilator use,[64] and bronchoconstriction after exercise in asthmatics and nonasthmatics.[22]

High levels of airborne nano/ultrafine PM have been identified at indoor ice rinks use fossil-fueled (gas, propane, or natural gas) Zambonis for ice resurfacing (**Fig. 4**)[65–67] and at athletic fields that are in close proximity to major roadways.[68] The prevalence of asthma and EIB in skating athletes has been documented to be between 20% and 50%. Several groups[69–71] evaluating elite figure skaters found that 29% to 35% tested positive for EIB by challenge test and Wilber and colleagues[71] reported that 50% of

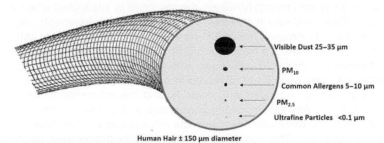

Visible Dust 25–35 μm

PM_{10}

Common Allergens 5–10 μm

$PM_{2.5}$

Ultrafine Particles <0.1 μm

Human Hair ± 150 μm diameter

Fig. 3. Particle diameters in relation to diameters of human hair, visible dust, and common allergens. PM, particulate matter.

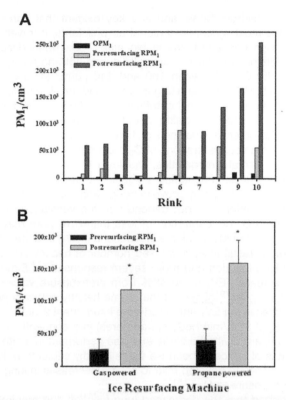

Fig. 4. (*A*) Comparing outside PM_1 (OPM) with preresurfacing and postresurfacing rink PM_1 (RPM) in 10 indoor ice rinks. The OPM values were from immediately outside each rink. (*B*) Comparing RPM between rinks serviced with gasoline-powered resurfacing machines (n = 6) with those using propane-powered resurfacing machines (n = 4). Differences between the preresurfacing and postresurfacing RPM_1 were evident within rinks ($P<.05$). Ice rinks resurfaced by fossil-fueled machines had higher baseline particulate levels, which became elevated during and immediately after each hourly resurfacing. (*From* Rundell KW. High levels of airborne ultrafine and fine particulate matter in indoor ice arenas. Inhal Toxicol 2003;15(3):237–50; with permission.)

female and 33% of male Olympic short track speed skaters and 25% of female long track speed skaters tested positive for EIB. Likewise, 21% of elite women ice hockey players tested positive for EIB[72] and showed a significant decrease in lung function over 4 years.[66] Exposure to high PM from fossil-fueled ice resurfacing machines during high ventilation exercise coupled with a genetic susceptibility could account for the observed high prevalence of asthma and EIB in ice rink athletes.[66,67,69–71]

Likewise, outdoor athletic fields and playgrounds in areas near high traffic roadways should be cause for concern because of traffic emissions. High levels of PM_1 (PM < 1 micrometer diameter) have been recorded at college soccer fields adjacent to major highways[68] and have been implicated in both acute[5,15,20–22,62] and chronic[66,72–74] effects on the pulmonary system.

Ozone

Ozone (O_3) is considered a secondary pollutant because it is formed from a photochemical reaction in atmosphere between nitrogen oxides, especially nitrogen dioxide

(NO_2), sunlight, and hydrocarbons, and is a key oxidant that can cause EIB.[75–77] Ozone is one of the most widespread global air pollutants; it travels with the wind, tending to reach high concentrations in big cities, downwind distant peripheries, and surrounding hills or mountains, especially during hot and sunny weather.[77] The current standards for O_3 is between 100 and 140 $\mu g/m^3$ (0.05–0.07 ppm) 8-hour mean, according to the World Health Organization and the US Environmental Protection Agency, respectively. Additional cutoffs include 160 $\mu g/m^3$ (0.08 ppm) that may affect health of susceptible exercising people, and a higher level of 240 $\mu g/m^3$ (0.12 ppm) defined as potentially having significant health effects, especially in vulnerable populations.[77] High concentrations of O_3 are a major problem in America and in Europe, and in hot climate megacities, the level of O_3 may exceed 400 $\mu g/m^3$ (0.20 ppm) for several days, constituting a significant threat to public health.[77]

Exercise in high levels of O_3 may provoke cough and substernal pain, and is correlated with O_3 concentration,[78,79] but depends on the ventilation rate and exercise duration. Although an O_3 concentration of less than 0.16 ppm may provoke small changes in the forced expiratory volume in 1 second (FEV_1) and forced vital capacity, higher concentrations result in an increased number of healthy subjects developing acute decreased lung function and more severe response.[78,79] Exposure to O_3 has been shown to decrease FEV_1 up to 48% from preexposure values.[79,80] Likewise, McDonnell and colleagues[79] observed that some healthy subjects without EIB had a 40% to 45% decrease in FEV_1 after moderate intermittent 2-hour exercise (ventilatory equivalent [VE] of 35 L/min/body surface area) in a concentration of O_3 greater than 0.24 ppm compared with the same exercise performed in a filtered air environment. This finding is of concern, because some healthy subjects without known EIB may be sensitive to O_3 and develop mild to severe decreases in lung function during a single exercise exposure to O_3.[79,81]

It is now recognized that the decreased lung function and respiratory symptoms from exercise in high [O_3] is primarily caused by stimulation of sensory nerves along conducting airways.[82–85] Inhaled O_3 reacts with epithelial fluid lining substrates, such as antioxidant molecules, membrane phospholipids, cholesterol, and macrophages to cause inflammatory mediator release and stimulation of airway sensory nerve endings.[86] The consequent release of neuropeptides, such as substance P, stimulates the axon reflex, which inhibits full inspiration, and causes reduced lung function and a rapid shallow breathing pattern.[87,88] The metabolites of cyclooxygenase-2 may in part mediate the stimulation of the nociceptive respiratory tract afferents and their inhibition may prevent the lung function changes owing to O_3.[89–92] Asthmatics with a lower baseline FEV_1 and uncontrolled asthma as well as susceptible healthy subjects may have an additional bronchoconstriction after exercise in O_3.[93]

Repeated daily exposure to O_3 combined with daily exercise periods causes a marked attenuation of discomfort from respiratory symptoms and the decreases in forced vital capacity and FEV_1 in a majority of subjects.[80,94–98] Some studies found no observable change in FEV_1 after O_3 exposure exercise, suggesting individual variability in the response to O_3.[99,100] In communities with high O_3 concentrations, the relative risk of developing asthma in children is related to time spend outside, and the number of outdoor sports played.[101] McConnell and colleagues[101] found that the relative risk of developing asthma in children playing 3 or more sports was 3.3 (95% confidence interval, 1.9–5.8), compared with children playing no sports in communities with high [O_3] or to children in areas of low O_3. Repeated episodes of O_3 inhalation may attenuate airway inflammation and neuropeptides release; rapid and shallow breathing occurs during the first days of exposure, and remodeling of the centriacinar airways is observed.[102] This finding suggests that O_3 exposure may contribute to the development of asthma and AHR in children and elite endurance summer sport athletes.

The O_3-induced bronchoconstriction may be partially reversed by albuterol.[103] Previous treatment with inhaled corticosteroids, or inhaled corticosteroids and long-acting beta agonists, does not prevent the neutrophilic airway inflammation or AHR owing to O_3 exposure in exercising mild asthmatics or healthy subjects who are susceptible to AHR.[104,105]

Nitrogen Dioxide

NO_2 is a reddish-brown gas with a characteristic pungent odor that can be noticeable during episodes of vehicular pollution. It is a key precursor of a range of secondary photochemically generated pollutants, such as ozone, and organic nitrate and sulfate particles measured as PM_{10} or $PM_{2.5}$. The major source of nitrogen oxides is from the combustion processes in stationary sources (power generation of the cities, heating) and in mobile sources (internal combustion, ie, vehicle emissions). Annual mean NO_2 concentrations in urban areas throughout the world are generally in the range of 20 to 90 μ/m^3 (0.01–0.05 ppm).[77] The World Health Organization standard levels for NO_2 are a 40 μ/m^3 (0.021 ppm) annual mean or a 200 μ/m^3 1-hour mean (0.106 ppm).[77] Hourly averages near very busy roads may exceed 940 μ/m^3 NO_2 (0.50 ppm).[77]

Mild asthmatics may be more susceptible to the potential effects of high [NO_2] than healthy subjects, with respect to airway responsiveness and lung function. In healthy subjects, short-term exposure of up to 2 hours, comprising periods of 10 to 30 minutes exercising at light to moderate intensity, does not provoke respiratory symptoms and shows no evidence of impaired pulmonary function when exposed to 0.12 to 4.00 ppm NO_2.[106–113] Mean airway narrowing after exercise does not seem to be different between filtered air or NO_2 inhaled during exercise in mild asthmatics.[109,112,114–118] However, similar to O_3, there is a great interindividual airway response to NO_2, especially in mild asthmatics.[119,120] NO_2 inhalation at [0.30 ppm] may potentiate EIB compared with a controlled exposure at similar workloads and ventilation rates.[119,120] Bauer and colleagues[119] observed a decrease in the FEV_1 of 9.4% after exercising for 10 minutes at a VE of 30 L/min in a filtered air environment, compared with a decrease of 37% when exercising with a concentration of 0.30 ppm of NO_2 in a particularly susceptible mild asthmatic who was treated with only short-acting beta agonists as needed. Jorres and Magnussen[114] observed that a mild asthmatic had a decrease in FEV_1 of 20%, whereas another had no change in FEV_1 after a 3-hour exposure to 1 ppm NO_2 while exercising for 10 minutes every 20 minutes at a VE of approximately 30 L/min.

Many studies have reported no increase in airway reactivity after exposure to NO_2,[114] whereas others found an increase in airway reactivity after low-dose exposure in the majority of mild asthmatics (0.10–0.20 ppm over 1–2 hours).[115,121] During a second day of exposure to 1 ppm NO_2 during 25 minutes of mild intensity exercise (2-fold the resting VE) every 30 minutes during a 2-hour period, Hackney and colleagues[122] observed an increase in respiratory symptoms despite finding no change in lung function. The increase in airway responsiveness after NO_2 exposure could be partially explained by the increase in thromboxane B_2, prostaglandin D_2, and various leukotrienes observed in mild asthmatics exposed to NO_2 while exercising, whereas 6ketoPGF1α, a metabolite of prostaglandin I_2 that is associated with bronchodilatation, was decreased in all subjects.[123] Sandstrom and colleagues[124] also noted a decrease in subset of lymphocytes after repeated exposure of 20 minutes NO_2, with 15 minutes of light exercise, possibly increasing susceptibility to airway infections.

This finding is of concern, especially in those with airway disease or athletes. Combined exposure to NO_2 and O_3 or PM does not seem to have additional or synergistic effects on airway function.[125,126]

Sulfur Dioxide

Sulfur dioxide (SO_2) is a gas originating from natural volcanic activity and industrial activities, such as the combustion of coal, petroleum, gasoline, and nondesulfurized natural gas.[77] The World Health Organization standards for SO_2 are 20 μ/m^3 (0.0075 ppm) for 24 hours or 500 μ/m^3 for a 10-minute mean (0.19 ppm).[77] Urban and rural concentrations are generally similar and the annual mean in European countries and is less than 50 $\mu g/m^3$ (0.019 ppm), with daily mean concentrations of less than 100 $\mu g/m^3$ (0.038 ppm). In the Baltimore, Maryland area, from June to September 2013, maximal 5-minute values of 229 ppb (600 μ/m^3) and 1-hour values of 134 ppb (351 μ/m^3) have been registered.[127] In the majority of healthy subjects, there are no significant effects on pulmonary function during exercise when exposed to SO_2 at ambient levels of less than 2 ppm, but exposure may accentuate the response to other pollutants such as O_3, especially in susceptible subjects, and when the concentration of both pollutants is high.[128–131] In asthmatics, SO_2 inhalation before or during exercise may elicit or aggravate bronchoconstriction and increase airway resistance at concentrations observed during ambient pollution episodes (0.4–0.6 ppm).[132–134] After a 10-minute exercise session with 1 ppm SO_2 exposure at a ventilation rate 6 times greater than resting values, asthmatics with EIB had a mean 23% decrease in FEV_1, whereas no change in pulmonary function was observed when exercising in filtered air.[135] Oronasal breathing of SO_2 during exercise may decrease the amplitude of response compared with oral breathing.[132,136] However, inhaled cromolyn or antileukotrienes has been shown to decrease SO_2-induced airway resistance and bronchoconstriction in asthmatics during exercise by preventing degranulation of airway mast cells and inhibiting the action of leukotrienes.[137,138]

Trichloramines

Trichloramines (NCl_3) belong to a family of byproducts from the reaction between chlorine disinfection products used in swimming pools and nitrogenous contaminants from swimmers, such as sweat, urine, soap residues, or cosmetics.[139–141] NCl_3 is the most volatile compound among the chloramines, is airborne at the water surface, and is strongly suspected to cause respiratory symptoms in swimmers. The characteristic chemical odor accompanying high levels of NCl_3 in the air[139,141] is often associated, in a dose–response manner, with the report of eye, nasal, and respiratory symptoms during training in swimmers, trainers, and lifeguards, and may trigger bronchoconstriction in asthmatics.[142–146] Although the high humidity conditions present at swimming pools are beneficial for asthmatics,[147] individuals should avoid swimming pools with a strong chlorine odor. The concentration of NCl_3 in swimming pool atmosphere is strongly dependent on the hygiene, activities of swimmers, water exchange rate, and swimming pool ventilation.[148] To avoid eye and respiratory tract infections, standards for chlorinated-disinfected swimming pool ambient air NCl_3 suggest not exceeding 0.3 to 0.5 mg/m^3.[145,148,149] However, NCl_3 is not routinely measured at most indoor swimming pools. Studies at municipal swimming pools in various countries report concentrations of NCl_3 in the atmosphere exceeding 0.5 mg/m^3,[3,150,151] despite within-standard levels in the water.

There is an association between regular indoor chlorinated pool attendance and the development of allergic diseases, bronchiolitis, and asthma in infants, young children, leisure adolescent swimmers, and adult swimmers,[152–166] but this relationship remains debatable.[167–169] Chronic exposure to chlorine N,N diethyl-1,4 phenylenedi-amine sulfate is responsible for occupational asthma in lifeguards and pool workers.[142,143,170,171] Recently, Rosenman and colleagues[171] reported that exposure to airborne chlorine byproducts by individuals who work at indoor swimming pools, water parks, or hydrotherapy spas was associated with the development of new onset asthma and triggering the EIB response in existing asthmatics.

The high-intensity exercise during swim training seems to be a major risk factor for the appearance of asthmatic symptoms.[172] In young competitive swimmers, the exercise load has been suggested to correlate with an increased AHR to histamine after swim training.[173] Years of NCl_3 exposure during repeated intense swimming sessions (ie, ≥ 10 h/wk) is implicated in development of atopy and allergies, AHR, and asthma in young adult competitive swimmers.[174–177] Bronchial biopsies from national-level competitive swimmers also showed similar airway remodeling and inflammation compared with mild asthmatic nonathletes, independent of airway responsiveness.[178] Because of a predominantly neutrophilic inflammation, corticosteroids may be ineffective in many swimmers.[179] Interestingly, this group does not typically have an exacerbation while swimming, likely because the high humidity at the pool surface provides a degree of protection. Castricum and colleagues[180] found that only 1 of 33 elite swimmers tested positive for EIB after an 8-minute swim challenge at an intensity of 85% or greater of the maximal heart rate, whereas 18 tested positive by a 6-minute dry air EVH challenge (**Fig. 5**), demonstrating the low asthmogenicity of swimming but high prevalence of EIB among this population.

Simultaneous Exposure to Multiple Environmental Triggers

It is clear that exposures to specific pollutants cause acute and chronic airway dysfunction, but it is also important to recognize that athletes are often simultaneously exposed to various combinations of each of these. For instance, the 20% to 50% prevalence of EIB reported in skaters far exceeds the approximate 8% to 12% prevalence in other athletes in the United States.[1,69–71] Chronic ventilation of the dry ice

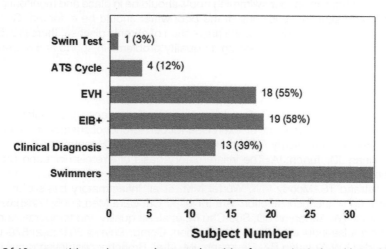

Fig. 5. Of 19 competitive swimmers who tested positive for exercise-induced bronchospasm (EIB), only 1 tested positive to a swim challenge test, likely owing to the high humidity at the water surface. (*Data from* Castricum A, Holzer K, Brukner P, et al. The role of the bronchial provocation challenge tests in the diagnosis of exercise-induced bronchoconstriction in elite swimmers. Br J Sports Med 2010;44(10):736–40.)

rink air by skating athletes during training and competition, coupled with high levels of PM_1 from fossil-fuel powered ice resurfacers, may exaggerate the EIB response, or directly cause airway damage that leads to new-onset asthma.[65] Ice rink air quality has been shown to be associated the high prevalence of airway dysfunction in skating athletes.[69,70] Likewise, urban athletic fields and school playgrounds can present a major health concern. College soccer players, both with and without a diagnosis of asthma, whose practice fields are in close proximity to major highways have shown significant decreases in lung function over the course of a season.[68]

SUMMARY AND PUBLIC HEALTH RECOMMENDATIONS

The prevalence of EIB and asthma among cold weather endurance athletes, ice rink sport athletes, and competitive swimmers is higher than in nonathletes and summer athletes, and has been related to repetitive inhalation of dry air and/or pollutants. In the United States, ozone, PM, and pool trichloramines are the pollutants most commonly encountered by training and competing athletes. Acute hyperpnoea of these pollutants during exercise have been shown to increase oxidative stress and trigger airway inflammation and decrease lung function. Acute effects on the respiratory system from pollution exposure have been documented in both the nonasthmatic and the asthmatic, with increased emergency department visits for respiratory distress during outbreaks of high pollution. Likewise, chronic exercise while breathing cold/dry air and/or these pollutants has been related to the development of new-onset asthma, EIB, and low resting lung function.

Despite the overwhelming evidence that air quality has a significant impact on respiratory health, many areas are not aware of the high ozone and PM that can be found at urban playgrounds and athletic fields along high traffic roadways and as such present a risk to young athletes. Only a few states do regulate where these recreation areas can be developed, and only 1 state does not allow the development of new athletic fields within 100 m of major highways; that particular state monitors ice rink pollution levels and allows only electric resurfacing in new rinks. Likewise, appropriate ventilation systems for indoor swimming pools should be in place and monitoring chlorine levels and sanitary conditions of the pool water should be enforced. Given the importance of exercise training for the prevention of chronic disease, there is substantial public health benefit in addressing air quality problems in sports and recreational areas.

REFERENCES

1. Weiler JM, Anderson SD, Randolph C, et al. Pathogenesis, prevalence, diagnosis, and management of exercise-induced bronchoconstriction: a practice parameter. Ann Allergy Asthma Immunol 2010;105(6 Suppl):S1–47.
2. Brannan JD, Turton JA. The inflammatory basis of exercise-induced bronchoconstriction. Phys Sportsmed 2010;38(4):67–73.
3. Hallstrand TS, Moody MW, Wurfel MM, et al. Inflammatory basis of exercise-induced bronchoconstriction. Am J Respir Crit Care Med 2005;172(6):679–86.
4. Rundell KW, Anderson SD, Sue-Chu M, et al. Air quality and temperature effects on exercise-induced bronchoconstriction. Compr Physiol 2015;5(2):579–610.
5. Rundell KW, Spiering BA, Baumann JM, et al. Bronchoconstriction provoked by exercise in a high-particulate-matter environment is attenuated by montelukast. Inhal Toxicol 2005;17(2):99–105.
6. Daigle CC, Chalupa DC, Gibb FR, et al. Ultrafine particle deposition in humans during rest and exercise. Inhal Toxicol 2003;15(6):539–52.

7. Cutrufello PT, Smoliga JM, Rundell KW. Small things make a big difference: particulate matter and exercise. Sports Med 2012;42(12):1041–58.

8. Zhang JJ, McCreanor JE, Cullinan P, et al. Health effects of real-world exposure to diesel exhaust in persons with asthma. Res Rep Health Eff Inst 2009;(138): 5–109 [discussion: 111–23].

9. McConnell R, Islam T, Shankardass K, et al. Childhood incident asthma and traffic-related air pollution at home and school. Environ Health Perspect 2010; 118(7):1021–6.

10. Islam T, McConnell R, Gauderman WJ, et al. Ozone, oxidant defense genes, and risk of asthma during adolescence. Am J Respir Crit Care Med 2008; 177(4):388–95.

11. Islam T, Gauderman WJ, Berhane K, et al. Relationship between air pollution, lung function and asthma in adolescents. Thorax 2007;62(11):957–63.

12. Jung KH, Torrone D, Lovinsky-Desir S, et al. Short-term exposure to PM2.5 and vanadium and changes in asthma gene DNA methylation and lung function decrements among urban children. Respir Res 2017;18(1):63.

13. Ciencewicki J, Trivedi S, Kleeberger SR. Oxidants and the pathogenesis of lung diseases. J Allergy Clin Immunol 2008;122(3):456–68 [quiz: 469–70].

14. Barreto M, Villa MP, Olita C, et al. 8-Isoprostane in exhaled breath condensate and exercise-induced bronchoconstriction in asthmatic children and adolescents. Chest 2009;135(1):66–73.

15. Rundell KW, Slee JB, Caviston R, et al. Decreased lung function after inhalation of ultrafine and fine particulate matter during exercise is related to decreased total nitrate in exhaled breath condensate. Inhal Toxicol 2008;20(1):1–9.

16. Barraza-Villarreal A, Sunyer J, Hernandez-Cadena L, et al. Air pollution, airway inflammation, and lung function in a cohort study of Mexico City schoolchildren. Environ Health Perspect 2008;116(6):832–8.

17. Chen BY, Chan CC, Lee CT, et al. The association of ambient air pollution with airway inflammation in schoolchildren. Am J Epidemiol 2012;175(8):764–74.

18. Salvi S, Blomberg A, Rudell B, et al. Acute inflammatory responses in the airways and peripheral blood after short-term exposure to diesel exhaust in healthy human volunteers. Am J Respir Crit Care Med 1999;159(3):702–9.

19. Salvi SS, Nordenhall C, Blomberg A, et al. Acute exposure to diesel exhaust increases IL-8 and GRO-alpha production in healthy human airways. Am J Respir Crit Care Med 2000;161(2 Pt 1):550–7.

20. Oberdorster G, Ferin J, Lehnert BE. Correlation between particle size, in vivo particle persistence, and lung injury. Environ Health Perspect 1994;102(Suppl 5):173–9.

21. Oberdorster G, Gelein RM, Ferin J, et al. Association of particulate air pollution and acute mortality: involvement of ultrafine particles? Inhal Toxicol 1995;7(1):111–24.

22. McCreanor J, Cullinan P, Nieuwenhuijsen MJ, et al. Respiratory effects of exposure to diesel traffic in persons with asthma. N Engl J Med 2007;357(23): 2348–58.

23. Nightingale JA, Maggs R, Cullinan P, et al. Airway inflammation after controlled exposure to diesel exhaust particulates. Am J Respir Crit Care Med 2000; 162(1):161–6.

24. Kelly FJ, Mudway I, Blomberg A, et al. Altered lung antioxidant status in patients with mild asthma. Lancet 1999;354(9177):482–3.

25. Zielinski H, Mudway IS, Berube KA, et al. Modeling the interactions of particulates with epithelial lining fluid antioxidants. Am J Physiol 1999;277(4 Pt 1): L719–26.

26. Mudway IS, Stenfors N, Duggan ST, et al. An in vitro and in vivo investigation of the effects of diesel exhaust on human airway lining fluid antioxidants. Arch Biochem Biophys 2004;423(1):200–12.

27. Rahman I, MacNee W. Oxidative stress and regulation of glutathione in lung inflammation. Eur Respir J 2000;16(3):534–54.

28. Ercan H, Birben E, Dizdar EA, et al. Oxidative stress and genetic and epidemiologic determinants of oxidant injury in childhood asthma. J Allergy Clin Immunol 2006;118(5):1097–104.

29. Hayes JD, McLellan LI. Glutathione and glutathione-dependent enzymes represent a co-ordinately regulated defence against oxidative stress. Free Radic Res 1999;31(4):273–300.

30. Islam T, Berhane K, McConnell R, et al. Glutathione-S-transferase (GST) P1, GSTM1, exercise, ozone and asthma incidence in school children. Thorax 2009;64(3):197–202.

31. Meyer A, Buhl R, Magnussen H. The effect of oral N-acetylcysteine on lung glutathione levels in idiopathic pulmonary fibrosis. Eur Respir J 1994;7(3):431–6.

32. Blesa S, Cortijo J, Martinez-Losa M, et al. Effectiveness of oral N-acetylcysteine in a rat experimental model of asthma. Pharmacol Res 2002;45(2):135–40.

33. Cortijo J, Marti-Cabrera M, de la Asuncion JG, et al. Contraction of human airways by oxidative stress protection by N-acetylcysteine. Free Radic Biol Med 1999;27(3–4):392–400.

34. Gillissen A, Nowak D. Characterization of N-acetylcysteine and ambroxol in antioxidant therapy. Respir Med 1998;92(4):609–23.

35. Kasielski M, Nowak D. Long-term administration of N-acetylcysteine decreases hydrogen peroxide exhalation in subjects with chronic obstructive pulmonary disease. Respir Med 2001;95(6):448–56.

36. Rubio ML, Martin-Mosquero MC, Ortega M, et al. Oral N-acetylcysteine attenuates elastase-induced pulmonary emphysema in rats. Chest 2004;125(4):1500–6.

37. Ginn-Pease ME, Whisler RL. Optimal NF kappa B mediated transcriptional responses in Jurkat T cells exposed to oxidative stress are dependent on intracellular glutathione and costimulatory signals. Biochem Biophys Res Commun 1996;226(3):695–702.

38. Wuyts WA, Vanaudenaerde BM, Dupont LJ, et al. N-acetylcysteine reduces chemokine release via inhibition of p38 MAPK in human airway smooth muscle cells. Eur Respir J 2003;22(1):43–9.

39. Koenig JQ, Mar TF, Allen RW, et al. Pulmonary effects of indoor- and outdoor-generated particles in children with asthma. Environ Health Perspect 2005; 113(4):499–503.

40. Radi R, Beckman JS, Bush KM, et al. Peroxynitrite-induced membrane lipid peroxidation: the cytotoxic potential of superoxide and nitric oxide. Arch Biochem Biophys 1991;288(2):481–7.

41. Pietropaoli AP, Frampton MW, Hyde RW, et al. Pulmonary function, diffusing capacity, and inflammation in healthy and asthmatic subjects exposed to ultrafine particles. Inhal Toxicol 2004;16(Suppl 1):59–72.

42. Henderson EM, Gaston B. SNOR and wheeze: the asthma enzyme? Trends Mol Med 2005;11(11):481–4.

43. Que LG, Liu L, Yan Y, et al. Protection from experimental asthma by an endogenous bronchodilator. Science 2005;308(5728):1618–21.

44. Zaman K, Hanigan MH, Smith A, et al. Endogenous S-nitrosoglutathione modifies 5-lipoxygenase expression in airway epithelial cells. Am J Respir Cell Mol Biol 2006;34(4):387–93.

45. Anderson SD, Daviskas E. The mechanism of exercise-induced asthma is....
    J Allergy Clin Immunol 2000;106(3):453–9.
46. Daviskas E, Gonda I, Anderson SD. Mathematical modeling of heat and
    water transport in human respiratory tract. J Appl Physiol (1985) 1990;
    69(1):362–72.
47. Anderson SD, Kippelen P. Airway injury as a mechanism for exercise-induced
    bronchoconstriction in elite athletes. J Allergy Clin Immunol 2008;122(2):
    225–35 [quiz: 236–7].
48. Strauss RH, McFadden ER Jr, Ingram RH Jr, et al. Influence of heat and humidity
    on the airway obstruction induced by exercise in asthma. J Clin Invest 1978;
    61(2):433–40.
49. Heir T, Oseid S. Self-reported asthma and exercise-induced asthma symptoms
    in high-level competitive cross-country skiers. Scand J Med Sci Sports 1994;
    4(2):128–33.
50. Larsson K, Ohlsen P, Larsson L, et al. High prevalence of asthma in cross coun-
    try skiers. BMJ 1993;307(6915):1326–9.
51. Karjalainen EM, Laitinen A, Sue-Chu M, et al. Evidence of airway inflammation
    and remodeling in ski athletes with and without bronchial hyperresponsiveness
    to methacholine. Am J Respir Crit Care Med 2000;161(6):2086–91.
52. Sue-Chu M, Larsson L, Moen T, et al. Bronchoscopy and bronchoalveolar
    lavage findings in cross-country skiers with and without "ski asthma". Eur Respir
    J 1999;13(3):626–32.
53. Sue-Chu M, Henriksen AH, Bjermer L. Non-invasive evaluation of lower airway
    inflammation in hyper-responsive elite cross-country skiers and asthmatics. Re-
    spir Med 1999;93(10):719–25.
54. Verges S, Floro P, Bianchi MP, et al. 10-year follow-up study of pulmonary func-
    tion in symptomatic elite cross-country skiers–athletes and bronchial dysfunc-
    tions. Scand J Med Sci Sports 2004;14(6):381–7.
55. Stensrud T, Berntsen S, Carlsen KH. Humidity influences exercise capacity in
    subjects with exercise-induced bronchoconstriction (EIB). Respir Med 2006;
    100(9):1633–41.
56. Price OJ, Hull JH, Backer V, et al. The impact of exercise-induced bronchocon-
    striction on athletic performance: a systematic review. Sports Med 2014;44(12):
    1749–61.
57. Kittelson DB, Watts WF, Johnson JP, et al. On-road exposure to highway aero-
    sols. 1. Aerosol and gas measurements. Inhal Toxicol 2004;16(Suppl 1):31–9.
58. Oberdorster G. Significance of particle parameters in the evaluation of
    exposure-dose-response relationships of inhaled particles. Inhal Toxicol 1996;
    8(Suppl):73–89.
59. Chalupa DC, Morrow PE, Oberdorster G, et al. Ultrafine particle deposition in
    subjects with asthma. Environ Health Perspect 2004;112(8):879–82.
60. Ware JH. Particulate air pollution and mortality–clearing the air. N Engl J Med
    2000;343(24):1798–9.
61. Werz O, Szellas D, Steinhilber D. Reactive oxygen species released from gran-
    ulocytes stimulate 5-lipoxygenase activity in a B-lymphocytic cell line. Eur J Bio-
    chem 2000;267(5):1263–9.
62. Atkinson RW, Anderson HR, Sunyer J, et al. Acute effects of particulate air pollu-
    tion on respiratory admissions: results from APHEA 2 project. Air pollution and
    health: a European approach. Am J Respir Crit Care Med 2001;164(10 Pt 1):
    1860–6.

63. Tolbert PE, Mulholland JA, MacIntosh DL, et al. Air quality and pediatric emergency room visits for asthma in Atlanta, Georgia, USA. Am J Epidemiol 2000; 151(8):798–810.
64. Hiltermann TJ, Stolk J, van der Zee SC, et al. Asthma severity and susceptibility to air pollution. Eur Respir J 1998;11(3):686–93.
65. Rundell KW. High levels of airborne ultrafine and fine particulate matter in indoor ice arenas. Inhal Toxicol 2003;15(3):237–50.
66. Rundell KW. Pulmonary function decay in women ice hockey players: is there a relationship to ice rink air quality? Inhal Toxicol 2004;16(3):117–23.
67. Rundell KW, Anderson SD, Spiering BA, et al. Field exercise vs laboratory eucapnic voluntary hyperventilation to identify airway hyperresponsiveness in elite cold weather athletes. Chest 2004;125(3):909–15.
68. Rundell KW, Caviston R, Hollenbach AM, et al. Vehicular air pollution, playgrounds, and youth athletic fields. Inhal Toxicol 2006;18(8):541–7.
69. Mannix ET, Farber MO, Palange P, et al. Exercise-induced asthma in figure skaters. Chest 1996;109(2):312–5.
70. Provost-Craig MA, Arbour KS, Sestili DC, et al. The incidence of exercise-induced bronchospasm in competitive figure skaters. J Asthma 1996;33(1): 67–71.
71. Wilber RL, Rundell KW, Szmedra L, et al. Incidence of exercise-induced bronchospasm in Olympic winter sport athletes. Med Sci Sports Exerc 2000;32(4): 732–7.
72. Rundell KW, Spiering BA, Evans TM, et al. Baseline lung function, exercise-induced bronchoconstriction, and asthma-like symptoms in elite women ice hockey players. Med Sci Sports Exerc 2004;36(3):405–10.
73. Gauderman WJ, Avol E, Gilliland F, et al. The effect of air pollution on lung development from 10 to 18 years of age. N Engl J Med 2004;351(11):1057–67.
74. McConnell R, Berhane K, Gilliland F, et al. Prospective study of air pollution and bronchitic symptoms in children with asthma. Am J Respir Crit Care Med 2003; 168(7):790–7.
75. Folinsbee LJ, Horstman DH, Kehrl HR, et al. Respiratory responses to repeated prolonged exposure to 0.12 ppm ozone. Am J Respir Crit Care Med 1994; 149(1):98–105.
76. Hazucha MJ, Folinsbee LJ, Bromberg PA. Distribution and reproducibility of spirometric response to ozone by gender and age. J Appl Physiol (1985) 2003;95(5):1917–25.
77. World Health Organization (WHO). WHO Air Quality Guidelines for particulate matter, ozone, nitrogen dioxide and sulfur dioxide. Denmark: Global Update; 2005.
78. Adams WC, Schelegle ES. Ozone and high ventilation effects on pulmonary function and endurance performance. J Appl Physiol Respir Environ Exerc Physiol 1983;55(3):805–12.
79. McDonnell WF, Horstman DH, Hazucha MJ, et al. Pulmonary effects of ozone exposure during exercise: dose-response characteristics. J Appl Physiol Respir Environ Exerc Physiol 1983;54(5):1345–52.
80. Horvath SM, Gliner JA, Folinsbee LJ. Adaptation to ozone: duration of effect. Am Rev Respir Dis 1981;123(5):496–9.
81. Balmes JR, Aris RM, Chen LL, et al. Effects of ozone on normal and potentially sensitive human subjects. Part I: airway inflammation and responsiveness to ozone in normal and asthmatic subjects. Res Rep Health Eff Inst 1997;(78): 1–37 [discussion: 81–99].

82. Adams WC. Effects of ozone exposure at ambient air pollution episode levels on exercise performance. Sports Med 1987;4(6):395–424.
83. Coleridge JC, Coleridge HM, Schelegle ES, et al. Acute inhalation of ozone stimulates bronchial C-fibers and rapidly adapting receptors in dogs. J Appl Physiol (1985) 1993;74(5):2345–52.
84. Hazucha MJ, Bates DV, Bromberg PA. Mechanism of action of ozone on the human lung. J Appl Physiol (1985) 1989;67(4):1535–41.
85. Krishna MT, Springall D, Meng QH, et al. Effects of ozone on epithelium and sensory nerves in the bronchial mucosa of healthy humans. Am J Respir Crit Care Med 1997;156(3 Pt 1):943–50.
86. Bromberg PA. Mechanisms of the acute effects of inhaled ozone in humans. Biochim Biophys Acta 2016;1860(12):2771–81.
87. Schelegle ES, Eldridge MW, Cross CE, et al. Differential effects of airway anesthesia on ozone-induced pulmonary responses in human subjects. Am J Respir Crit Care Med 2001;163(5):1121–7.
88. Vesely KR, Schelegle ES, Stovall MY, et al. Breathing pattern response and epithelial labeling in ozone-induced airway injury in neutrophil-depleted rats. Am J Respir Cell Mol Biol 1999;20(4):699–709.
89. Alexis N, Urch B, Tarlo S, et al. Cyclooxygenase metabolites play a different role in ozone-induced pulmonary function decline in asthmatics compared to normals. Inhal Toxicol 2000;12(12):1205–24.
90. Hazucha MJ, Madden M, Pape G, et al. Effects of cyclo-oxygenase inhibition on ozone-induced respiratory inflammation and lung function changes. Eur J Appl Physiol Occup Physiol 1996;73(1–2):17–27.
91. Schelegle ES, Adams WC, Siefkin AD. Indomethacin pretreatment reduces ozone-induced pulmonary function decrements in human subjects. Am Rev Respir Dis 1987;136(6):1350–4.
92. Ying RL, Gross KB, Terzo TS, et al. Indomethacin does not inhibit the ozone-induced increase in bronchial responsiveness in human subjects. Am Rev Respir Dis 1990;142(4):817–21.
93. Horstman DH, Ball BA, Brown J, et al. Comparison of pulmonary responses of asthmatic and nonasthmatic subjects performing light exercise while exposed to a low level of ozone. Toxicol Ind Health 1995;11(4):369–85.
94. Farrell BP, Kerr HD, Kulle TJ, et al. Adaptation in human subjects to the effects of inhaled ozone after repeated exposure. Am Rev Respir Dis 1979;119(5):725–30.
95. Folinsbee LJ, Bedi JF, Horvath SM. Respiratory responses in humans repeatedly exposed to low concentrations of ozone. Am Rev Respir Dis 1980;121(3):431–9.
96. Hackney JD, Linn WS, Mohler JG, et al. Adaptation to short-term respiratory effects of ozone in men exposed repeatedly. J Appl Physiol Respir Environ Exerc Physiol 1977;43(1):82–5.
97. Kulle TJ, Sauder LR, Kerr HD, et al. Duration of pulmonary function adaptation to ozone in humans. Am Ind Hyg Assoc J 1982;43(11):832–7.
98. Linn WS, Medway DA, Anzar UT, et al. Persistence of adaptation to ozone in volunteers exposed repeatedly for six weeks. Am Rev Respir Dis 1982;125(5):491–5.
99. Foxcroft WJ, Adams WC. Effects of ozone exposure on four consecutive days on work performance and VO2max. J Appl Physiol (1985) 1986;61(3):960–6.
100. Gliner JA, Horvath SM, Folinsbee LJ. Preexposure to low ozone concentrations does not diminish the pulmonary function response on exposure to higher ozone concentrations. Am Rev Respir Dis 1983;127(1):51–5.

101. McConnell R, Berhane K, Gilliland F, et al. Asthma in exercising children exposed to ozone: a cohort study. Lancet 2002;359(9304):386–91.
102. Schelegle ES, Walby WF, Alfaro MF, et al. Repeated episodes of ozone inhalation attenuates airway injury/repair and release of substance P, but not adaptation. Toxicol Appl Pharmacol 2003;186(3):127–42.
103. Beckett WS, McDonnell WF, Horstman DH, et al. Role of the parasympathetic nervous system in acute lung response to ozone. J Appl Physiol (1985) 1985;59(6):1879–85.
104. Nightingale JA, Rogers DF, Chung KF, et al. No effect of inhaled budesonide on the response to inhaled ozone in normal subjects. Am J Respir Crit Care Med 2000;161(2 Pt 1):479–86.
105. Vagaggini B, Bartoli ML, Cianchetti S, et al. Increase in markers of airway inflammation after ozone exposure can be observed also in stable treated asthmatics with minimal functional response to ozone. Respir Res 2010;11:5.
106. Bylin G, Lindvall T, Rehn T, et al. Effects of short-term exposure to ambient nitrogen dioxide concentrations on human bronchial reactivity and lung function. Eur J Respir Dis 1985;66(3):205–17.
107. Folinsbee LJ, Horvath SM, Bedi JF, et al. Effect of 0.62 ppm NO2 on cardiopulmonary function in young male nonsmokers. Environ Res 1978;15(2):199–205.
108. Frampton MW, Morrow PE, Cox C, et al. Effects of nitrogen dioxide exposure on pulmonary function and airway reactivity in normal humans. Am Rev Respir Dis 1991;143(3):522–7.
109. Kerr HD, Kulle TJ, McIlhany ML, et al. Effects of nitrogen dioxide on pulmonary function in human subjects: an environmental chamber study. Environ Res 1979;19(2):392–404.
110. Kim SU, Koenig JQ, Pierson WE, et al. Acute pulmonary effects of nitrogen dioxide exposure during exercise in competitive athletes. Chest 1991;99(4):815–9.
111. Koenig JQ, Covert DS, Smith MS, et al. The pulmonary effects of ozone and nitrogen dioxide alone and combined in healthy and asthmatic adolescent subjects. Toxicol Ind Health 1988;4(4):521–32.
112. Linn WS, Solomon JC, Trim SC, et al. Effects of exposure to 4 ppm nitrogen dioxide in healthy and asthmatic volunteers. Arch Environ Health 1985;40(4):234–9.
113. Azadniv M, Utell MJ, Morrow PE, et al. Effects of nitrogen dioxide exposure on human host defense. Inhal Toxicol 1998;10(6):585–601.
114. Jorres R, Magnussen H. Effect of 0.25 ppm nitrogen dioxide on the airway response to methacholine in asymptomatic asthmatic patients. Lung 1991;169(2):77–85.
115. Kleinman MT, Bailey RM, Linn WS, et al. Effects of 0.2 ppm nitrogen dioxide on pulmonary function and response to bronchoprovocation in asthmatics. J Toxicol Environ Health 1983;12(4–6):815–26.
116. Koenig JQ, Covert DS, Marshall SG, et al. The effects of ozone and nitrogen dioxide on pulmonary function in healthy and in asthmatic adolescents. Am Rev Respir Dis 1987;136(5):1152–7.
117. Linn WS, Shamoo DA, Avol EL, et al. Dose-response study of asthmatic volunteers exposed to nitrogen dioxide during intermittent exercise. Arch Environ Health 1986;41(5):292–6.
118. Rubinstein I, Bigby BG, Reiss TF, et al. Short-term exposure to 0.3 ppm nitrogen dioxide does not potentiate airway responsiveness to sulfur dioxide in asthmatic subjects. Am Rev Respir Dis 1990;141(2):381–5.

119. Bauer MA, Utell MJ, Morrow PE, et al. Inhalation of 0.30 ppm nitrogen dioxide potentiates exercise-induced bronchospasm in asthmatics. Am Rev Respir Dis 1986;134(6):1203–8.
120. Roger LJ, Horstman DH, McDonnell W, et al. Pulmonary function, airway responsiveness, and respiratory symptoms in asthmatics following exercise in NO2. Toxicol Ind Health 1990;6(1):155–71.
121. Orehek J, Massari JP, Gayrard P, et al. Effect of short-term, low-level nitrogen dioxide exposure on bronchial sensitivity of asthmatic patients. J Clin Invest 1976;57(2):301–7.
122. Hackney JD, Thiede FC, Linn WS, et al. Experimental studies on human health effects of air pollutants. IV. Short-term physiological and clinical effects of nitrogen dioxide exposure. Arch Environ Health 1978;33(4):176–80.
123. Jorres R, Nowak D, Grimminger F, et al. The effect of 1 ppm nitrogen dioxide on bronchoalveolar lavage cells and inflammatory mediators in normal and asthmatic subjects. Eur Respir J 1995;8(3):416–24.
124. Sandstrom T, Helleday R, Bjermer L, et al. Effects of repeated exposure to 4 ppm nitrogen dioxide on bronchoalveolar lymphocyte subsets and macrophages in healthy men. Eur Respir J 1992;5(9):1092–6.
125. Folinsbee LJ, Bedi JF, Horvath SM. Combined effects of ozone and nitrogen dioxide on respiratory function in man. Am Ind Hyg Assoc J 1981;42(7):534–41.
126. Koenig JQ, Covert DS, Morgan MS, et al. Acute effects of 0.12 ppm ozone or 0.12 ppm nitrogen dioxide on pulmonary function in healthy and asthmatic adolescents. Am Rev Respir Dis 1985;132(3):648–51.
127. Shepherd MA, Haynatzki G, Rautiainen R, et al. Estimates of community exposure and health risk to sulfur dioxide from power plant emissions using short-term mobile and stationary ambient air monitoring. J Air Waste Manag Assoc 2015;65(10):1239–46.
128. Bedi JF, Folinsbee LJ, Horvath SM, et al. Human exposure to sulfur dioxide and ozone: absence of a synergistic effect. Arch Environ Health 1979;34(4):233–9.
129. Folinsbee LJ, Bedi JF, Horvath SM. Pulmonary response to threshold levels of sulfur dioxide (1.0 ppm) and ozone (0.3 ppm). J Appl Physiol (1985) 1985;58(6):1783–7.
130. Hazucha M, Bates DV. Combined effect of ozone and sulphur dioxide on human pulmonary function. Nature 1975;257(5521):50–1.
131. van Thriel C, Schaper M, Kleinbeck S, et al. Sensory and pulmonary effects of acute exposure to sulfur dioxide (SO2). Toxicol Lett 2010;196(1):42–50.
132. Kirkpatrick MB, Sheppard D, Nadel JA, et al. Effect of the oronasal breathing route on sulfur dioxide-induced bronchoconstriction in exercising asthmatic subjects. Am Rev Respir Dis 1982;125(6):627–31.
133. Linn WS, Venet TG, Shamoo DA, et al. Respiratory effects of sulfur dioxide in heavily exercising asthmatics. A dose-response study. Am Rev Respir Dis 1983;127(3):278–83.
134. Sheppard D, Saisho A, Nadel JA, et al. Exercise increases sulfur dioxide-induced bronchoconstriction in asthmatic subjects. Am Rev Respir Dis 1981;123(5):486–91.
135. Koenig JQ, Pierson WE, Horike M, et al. Effects of SO2 plus NaCl aerosol combined with moderate exercise on pulmonary function in asthmatic adolescents. Environ Res 1981;25(2):340–8.
136. Linn WS, Shamoo DA, Spier CE, et al. Respiratory effects of 0.75 ppm sulfur dioxide in exercising asthmatics: influence of upper-respiratory defenses. Environ Res 1983;30(2):340–8.

137. Gong H Jr, Linn WS, Terrell SL, et al. Anti-inflammatory and lung function effects of montelukast in asthmatic volunteers exposed to sulfur dioxide. Chest 2001; 119(2):402–8.

138. Sheppard D, Nadel JA, Boushey HA. Inhibition of sulfur dioxide-induced bronchoconstriction by disodium cromoglycate in asthmatic subjects. Am Rev Respir Dis 1981;124(3):257–9.

139. Florentin A, Hautemaniere A, Hartemann P. Health effects of disinfection by-products in chlorinated swimming pools. Int J Hyg Environ Health 2011; 214(6):461–9.

140. Keuten MG, Schets FM, Schijven JF, et al. Definition and quantification of initial anthropogenic pollutant release in swimming pools. Water Res 2012;46(11): 3682–92.

141. World Health Organization (WHO). International programme on chemical safety, environmental health criteria 216: disinfectants and disinfectant by-products. Geneva (Switzerland): World Health Organization; 2000.

142. Fantuzzi G, Righi E, Predieri G, et al. Airborne trichloramine (NCl(3)) levels and self-reported health symptoms in indoor swimming pool workers: dose-response relationships. J Expo Sci Environ Epidemiol 2013;23(1):88–93.

143. Jacobs JH, Spaan S, van Rooy GB, et al. Exposure to trichloramine and respiratory symptoms in indoor swimming pool workers. Eur Respir J 2007;29(4): 690–8.

144. Levesque B, Duchesne JF, Gingras S, et al. The determinants of prevalence of health complaints among young competitive swimmers. Int Arch Occup Environ Health 2006;80(1):32–9.

145. Parrat J, Donze G, Iseli C, et al. Assessment of occupational and public exposure to trichloramine in Swiss indoor swimming pools: a proposal for an occupational exposure limit. Ann Occup Hyg 2012;56(3):264–77.

146. Potts JE. Adverse respiratory health effects of competitive swimming: the prevalence of symptoms, illnesses, and bronchial responsiveness to methacholine and exercise. University of British Columbia; 1994.

147. Fitch KD, Morton AR, Blanksby BA. Effects of swimming training on children with asthma. Arch Dis Child 1976;51(3):190–4.

148. Levesque B, Vezina L, Gauvin D, et al. Investigation of air quality problems in an indoor swimming pool: a case study. Ann Occup Hyg 2015;59(8):1085–9.

149. World Health Organization (WHO). WHO Guidelines for safe recreational water environments: swimming pools and similar environments. vol. 2. Geneva: World Health Organization; 2006.

150. Seys SF, Feyen L, Keirsbilck S, et al. An outbreak of swimming-pool related respiratory symptoms: an elusive source of trichloramine in a municipal indoor swimming pool. Int J Hyg Environ Health 2015;218(4):386–91.

151. Zare Afifi M, Blatchley ER 3rd. Seasonal dynamics of water and air chemistry in an indoor chlorinated swimming pool. Water Res 2015;68:771–83.

152. Bernard A, Carbonnelle S, de Burbure C, et al. Chlorinated pool attendance, atopy, and the risk of asthma during childhood. Environ Health Perspect 2006;114(10):1567–73.

153. Bernard A, Nickmilder M, Voisin C. Outdoor swimming pools and the risks of asthma and allergies during adolescence. Eur Respir J 2008;32(4):979–88.

154. Bernard A, Nickmilder M, Voisin C, et al. Impact of chlorinated swimming pool attendance on the respiratory health of adolescents. Pediatrics 2009;124(4): 1110–8.

155. Bernard A, Voisin C, Sardella A. Con: respiratory risks associated with chlorinated swimming pools: a complex pattern of exposure and effects. Am J Respir Crit Care Med 2011;183(5):570–2.
156. Chaumont A, Voisin C, Sardella A, et al. Interactions between domestic water hardness, infant swimming and atopy in the development of childhood eczema. Environ Res 2012;116:52–7.
157. Ferrari M, Schenk K, Mantovani W, et al. Attendance at chlorinated indoor pools and risk of asthma in adult recreational swimmers. J Sci Med Sport 2011;14(3):184–9.
158. Font-Ribera L, Kogevinas M, Zock JP, et al. Swimming pool attendance and risk of asthma and allergic symptoms in children. Eur Respir J 2009;34(6):1304–10.
159. Jacobs JH, Fuertes E, Krop EJ, et al. Swimming pool attendance and respiratory symptoms and allergies among Dutch children. Occup Environ Med 2012;69(11):823–30.
160. Kogevinas M, Villanueva CM, Font-Ribera L, et al. Genotoxic effects in swimmers exposed to disinfection by-products in indoor swimming pools. Environ Health Perspect 2010;118(11):1531–7.
161. Kohlhammer Y, Doring A, Schafer T, et al. Swimming pool attendance and hay fever rates later in life. Allergy 2006;61(11):1305–9.
162. Nickmilder M, Bernard A. Ecological association between childhood asthma and availability of indoor chlorinated swimming pools in Europe. Occup Environ Med 2007;64(1):37–46.
163. Schoefer Y, Zutavern A, Brockow I, et al. Health risks of early swimming pool attendance. Int J Hyg Environ Health 2008;211(3–4):367–73.
164. Voisin C, Sardella A, Marcucci F, et al. Infant swimming in chlorinated pools and the risks of bronchiolitis, asthma and allergy. Eur Respir J 2010;36(1):41–7.
165. Weisel CP, Richardson SD, Nemery B, et al. Childhood asthma and environmental exposures at swimming pools: state of the science and research recommendations. Environ Health Perspect 2009;117(4):500–7.
166. Bernard A, Carbonnelle S, Dumont X, et al. Infant swimming practice, pulmonary epithelium integrity, and the risk of allergic and respiratory diseases later in childhood. Pediatrics 2007;119(6):1095–103.
167. Font-Ribera L, Villanueva CM, Nieuwenhuijsen MJ, et al. Swimming pool attendance, asthma, allergies, and lung function in the Avon Longitudinal Study of Parents and Children cohort. Am J Respir Crit Care Med 2011;183(5):582–8.
168. Piacentini GL, Baraldi E. Pro: swimming in chlorinated pools and risk of asthma: we can now carry on sending our children to swimming pools! Am J Respir Crit Care Med 2011;183(5):569–70.
169. Valeriani F, Protano C, Vitali M, et al. Swimming attendance during childhood and development of asthma: meta-analysis. Pediatr Int 2017;59(7):846–7.
170. Demange V, Bohadana A, Massin N, et al. Exhaled nitric oxide and airway hyperresponsiveness in workers: a preliminary study in lifeguards. BMC Pulm Med 2009;9:53.
171. Rosenman KD, Millerick-May M, Reilly MJ, et al. Swimming facilities and work-related asthma. J Asthma 2015;52(1):52–8.
172. Paivinen MK, Keskinen KL, Tikkanen HO. Swimming and asthma: factors underlying respiratory symptoms in competitive swimmers. Clin Respir J 2010;4(2):97–103.
173. Carlsen KH, Oseid S, Odden H. The response of children with and without bronchial asthma to heavy swimming exercise. In: Oseid S, Carlsen KH, editors. Children and exercise. Champaign (IL): Human Kinetics; 1989. p. 351–60.

174. Bougault V, Boulet LP. Airways disorders and the swimming pool. Immunol Allergy Clin North Am 2013;33(3):395–408, ix.
175. Bougault V, Turmel J, Boulet LP. Bronchial challenges and respiratory symptoms in elite swimmers and winter sport athletes: airway hyperresponsiveness in asthma: its measurement and clinical significance. Chest 2010;138(2 Suppl): 31s–7s.
176. Helenius IJ, Tikkanen HO, Sarna S, et al. Asthma and increased bronchial responsiveness in elite athletes: atopy and sport event as risk factors. J Allergy Clin Immunol 1998;101(5):646–52.
177. Bernard A. Chlorination products: emerging links with allergic diseases. Curr Med Chem 2007;14(16):1771–82.
178. Bougault V, Loubaki L, Joubert P, et al. Airway remodeling and inflammation in competitive swimmers training in indoor chlorinated swimming pools. J Allergy Clin Immunol 2012;129(2):351–8, 358.e1.
179. Gelardi M, Ventura MT, Fiorella R, et al. Allergic and non-allergic rhinitis in swimmers: clinical and cytological aspects. Br J Sports Med 2012;46(1):54–8.
180. Castricum A, Holzer K, Brukner P, et al. The role of the bronchial provocation challenge tests in the diagnosis of exercise-induced bronchoconstriction in elite swimmers. Br J Sports Med 2010;44(10):736–40.

Exercise-Induced Bronchoconstriction
Background, Prevalence, and Sport Considerations

Matteo Bonini, MD, PhD[a],*, William Silvers, MD[b]

KEYWORDS

- Asthma • Bronchoconstriction • Exercise • Athlete • Prevalence • Sport discipline

KEY POINTS

- Exercise-induced bronchoconstriction (EIB) is defined as the transient airway narrowing that occurs as a result of exercise.
- Current guidelines recommend distinguishing EIB with underlying clinical asthma from the occurrence of exercise-induced bronchial obstruction in subjects without other symptoms and signs of asthma.
- EIB has been reported in up to 90% of asthmatic patients, reflecting the level of disease control, but it may develop even in subjects without clinical asthma, particularly in athletes, children, subjects with atopy or rhinitis, and following respiratory infections.
- The intensity, duration, and type of training have been associated with the occurrence of EIB with higher prevalence rates in endurance sports, winter disciplines, and swimming.
- When properly managed, EIB does not restrict exercise performance and does not prevent competition at elite level.

BACKGROUND

Regular physical activity is strongly recommended by all principal health care systems and evidence-based guidelines as one of the most effective means to prevent chronic diseases and maintain good health.[1] Indeed, extensive evidence exists regarding the beneficial effect of training and rehabilitation programs in respiratory diseases, including asthma.[2] It has been shown that physical activity can improve symptoms, quality of life, exercise capacity, and pulmonary function, as well as reduce airway inflammation and responsiveness in asthmatic subjects.[3–5]

Disclosure Statement: The authors have no conflict of interest to declare.
[a] Airways Disease Section, National Heart and Lung Institute (NHLI), Royal Brompton Hospital, Imperial College London, Dovehouse Street, London SW3 6LY, UK; [b] University of Colorado School of Medicine, 13001 E 17th Place, Aurora, CO 80045, USA
* Corresponding author.
E-mail address: m.bonini@imperial.ac.uk

On the other hand, vigorous physical training may trigger airway symptoms by imposing high demands on the respiratory system and by exposing subjects to increased amounts of inhalant allergens, pollutants, irritants, and adverse environmental conditions.[6] Furthermore, intense physical training may induce a transient status of immune downregulation with a shift toward a prevalent T-lymphocyte helper-2 response, clinically associated with an increased prevalence of atopy and viral upper respiratory tract infections, both representing relevant risk factors for the onset and worsening of asthma.[7,8]

The transient airway narrowing that occurs as a result of exercise is defined exercise-induced bronchoconstriction (EIB).[6] Already in the first century AD, Araeteus the Cappadocian described respiratory symptoms induced by physical exercise: "if from running, gymnastics, or any other work, breathing becomes difficult, it is called asthma."[9] However, a scientific objective interest for this phenomenon can be dated back to 1960, when Jones and coworkers[10] focused on the physiologic response to exercise in asthmatic children and named the airway obstruction after an exercise challenge "exercise-induced asthma" (EIA). Subsequent studies defined the different patterns of response to exercise in asthmatic patients, the effect of type, intensity, and duration of challenges, and the influence of antiasthmatic drugs on EIA.[11] In reviewing these findings, Godfrey[12] concluded that "despite of some exceptions, there has been no evidence that EIA occurs in patients other than asthmatics, and although sporadic cases have been reported where exercise appears to have been the only precipitant of asthma in a patient, careful investigation has usually revealed other clinical and physiological manifestations of bronchial asthma." Although some investigators consider EIA a distinct asthma phenotype,[13] it is quite evident that exercise may trigger bronchial obstruction and clinical symptoms in almost all asthmatic patients, independently from the underlying causes and mechanisms of asthma.[14] However, the concept that exercise may induce bronchial obstruction only in asthmatic patients is currently under debate.[15] In fact, despite the physiologic response to exercise, which usually results in slight bronchodilation, EIB may develop even in subjects without clinical asthma.[9] To bring some clarity to this still controversial issue, a Practice Parameter, jointly developed by the American Academy/College of Allergy Asthma and Immunology,[16] recommended to abandon the term of EIA, and more recently, an American Thoracic Society Clinical Practice Guideline[6] suggests naming EIB with asthma (EIBa), the occurrence of bronchial obstruction after exercise in asthmatic patients, and EIB without asthma (EIBwa), the occurrence of EIB in subjects without other symptoms and signs of clinical asthma.

EIB typically develops within 15 minutes following at least 5 to 8 minutes of high-intensity aerobic training (>85% of maximal voluntary ventilation), although it can also occur during exercise, and spontaneously resolves within 60 minutes.[17] After an episode of EIB, there is often a refractory period of about 1 to 3 hours during which, if exercise is repeated, the bronchoconstriction is less accentuated.[12] The increase in airway osmolarity due to the respiratory water loss and the vasodilation associated with airways rewarming has been reported to be the major determinants of EIB (osmotic and thermal theories).[18,19] Furthermore, a direct damage of the bronchial epithelium caused by viral infections, occupational agents and exercise, as well as an autonomic dysregulation may represent alternative causal mechanisms.[11] Most common symptoms include cough, dyspnea, breathlessness, wheezing, and chest tightness.[6] A careful history taking and physical examination is always recommended.[20] The use of specific questionnaires for screening allergic and respiratory diseases in athletes and exercisers represents a useful and easy-to-use additional diagnostic tool.[21] However, research performed over the years has consistently shown a poor relationship between the presence of "asthmalike" symptoms and objective evidence of EIB.[22] Furthermore, pulmonary function tests at baseline seem to be poorly predictive of EIB in athletes, often being within the normal ranges even in the presence of disease.[23] Thus, in order to establish a secure diagnosis of EIB, it is critical to perform objective testing to confirm dynamic changes in airway function.[6,24] The differential diagnosis of EIB should take into account several entities, such as physiologic exercise limitations, exercise-induced laryngeal dysfunctions, exercise-induced anaphylaxis, and shortness of breath with exercise due to lung diseases (other than asthma), and metabolic and cardiac diseases.[6,25,26] Management of EIB includes multiple effective pharmacologic and nonpharmacologic strategies,[6,17,27] but should take into high consideration onset of tolerance,[28] side effects,[29] and, in elite athletes, anti–doping regulations.[30]

PREVALENCE

The prevalence of EIB varies from 5% to 20% in the general population and has been reported to be up to 90% in asthmatic subjects, reflecting the level of disease control, with EIBa occurring more frequently in more severe and uncontrolled asthmatic patients.[14] EIBwa is also particularly frequent in athletes,[31] children,[32,33] subjects with rhinitis,[34] and following respiratory infections.[35]

In particular, several studies called attention to an increased occurrence of asthma and EIB in athletes, with prevalence rates widely ranging from 3.7% to 54.8% (**Table 1**) depending on the study population and the criteria used for diagnosis (ie, questionnaires, anti–doping records, baseline spirometry, bronchial provocation challenges). Independently from these potential confounders, studies performed in comparable samples and with similar diagnostic methodologies seem to indicate that the asthma incidence is on the increase: from 9.7% in 1976 to 11.2% in 1984, 16.7% in 1996 and 21.0% in 2000 in the US Olympic delegation.[36–38] More recently, a 12-year study including 4 cross-sectional surveys performed between 2000 and 2012, before Summer and Winter Olympics, showed that the prevalence of asthma in 659 Italian Olympic athletes was 14.7%, with a significant increase from 2000 (11.3%) to 2008 (17.2%).

With regards to a gender effect,[39] a study recently performed in 187 elite athletes (101 swimmers and 86 tennis players) showed a higher prevalence of asthma symptoms in women, although there was no significant difference in the prevalence of EIB when measured through a mannitol and a sport-specific challenge.[40] Norqvist and colleagues[41] also reported that, compared with men, elite female athletes had a higher prevalence of asthma, respiratory symptoms, use of medications, and health care services.

It has been also extensively reported that asthma and allergic rhinitis frequently coexist, with symptoms of rhinitis being reported in 80% to 90% of asthma patients, and asthma symptoms reported in 20% to 40% of patients with allergic rhinitis.[34] Prospective studies also suggest that rhinitis frequently precedes the development of asthma[42] and that many patients with rhinitis alone show nonspecific bronchial hyperresponsiveness after exercise or methacholine, this being a risk factor for developing asthma.[43] Furthermore, it has been proven that the severity of allergic rhinitis and asthma is related and that proper management of allergic rhinitis improves asthma control.[34] In addition, exercise can be a trigger for rhinitis, especially in outdoor sports and even greater with cold dry air exposure in winter sports, for example, the "skier's nose."[44] On the basis of all the above, the Alergic Rhinitis and its Impact on Asthma (ARIA) recommendation[34] to screen every subject with rhinitis for asthma should be also extended to athletes.[45]

Table 1
Prevalence of asthma and exercise-induced bronchoconstriction among athletes

Type of Sport	Study Population (n)	Prevalence, %	Methodology for Diagnosis	Reference
Olympic teams	US 1998 Olympic team (170)	23.0	Spirometry, exercise challenge	Wilber, 2000
	US 1998 Olympic team (196)	21.9	Questionnaire	Weiler, 2000
	Australian 2000 Olympic team (214)	21.0	Questionnaire	Katelaris et al,[38] 2000
	US 1996 Olympic team (699)	16.7	Questionnaire	Weiler et al,[37] 1998
	Italian Olympic athletes (659)	14.7	Questionnaires, lung function tests	Bonini et al,[11] 2015
	Polish 2008 Olympic team (222)	11.3	Questionnaire, spirometry, methacholine challenge	Kurowski, 2016
	US 1984 Olympic team (597)	11.2	Questionnaire, exercise challenge	Voy,[36] 1984
	Italian 2000 pre-Olympic team (265)	10.9	Questionnaire, spirometry	Lapucci, 2003
	Australian 1976 Olympic team (185)	9.7	Physical examination	Fitch, 1984
	Australian 1980 Olympic team (106)	8.5	Physical examination	Fitch, 1984
	Spanish 1982 Olympic team (495)	4.4	Questionnaire	Drobnic, 1994
Winter sports	Cross-country skiers (42)	54.8	Questionnaire, spirometry, methacholine challenge	Larsson et al,[54] 1993
	Swedish and Norwegian cross-country skiers (171)	42.0/12.0	Questionnaire, spirometry, methacholine challenge	Sue-Chu et al,[55] 1996
	Ice hockey players (88)	21.5	Questionnaire, spirometry, histamine challenge	Lumme, 2003
	Ice hockey players (50)	11.5	Questionnaire, spirometry, methacholine and exercise challenge	Leuppi, 1998
	Cross-country skiers (20)	10.0	Exercise challenge	Pohjantähti, 2005
Swimming	Swimmers (90)	39.0	EVH challenge	Bougault, 2010
	US swimmers (738)	13.4	Questionnaire	Potts, 1996
Track and field	Marathon runners (208)	32.0	Questionnaire	Robson-Ansley et al,[51] 2012
	Finnish runners (103)	15.5	Questionnaire	Tikkanen, 1994

(continued on next page)

Table 1
(continued)

Type of Sport	Study Population (n)	Prevalence, %	Methodology for Diagnosis	Reference
Various sports	US college athletes (80)	42.5	Questionnaire, exercise challenge	Burnett, 2016
	Summer athletes (162)	22.8	Questionnaire, spirometry, histamine challenge	Helenius et al,[70] 1998
	Swiss athletes (2060)	3.7	Questionnaire	Helbling, 1990
	Figure skaters (124)	35.0	Exercise challenge	Mannix, 1996
	US football players (151)	50.6	Questionnaire, methacholine challenge	Weiler, 1986

Despite extensive epidemiologic data, EIB evolution in athletes has not been yet fully studied. However, in athletes who stopped intensive training, EIB attenuated or even disappeared, whereas symptoms and airway inflammation increased among those who remained active during the follow-up period, irrespective of treatment strategies. Thus, EIB in athletes seems to be only partly reversible, and active training appears to be a causative factor of airway inflammation and symptoms.[46]

SPORT CONSIDERATIONS

The intensity, duration, and type of training have been associated with the occurrence of bronchial symptoms, airway hyperresponsiveness, and asthma in elite athletes (Table 2).

Table 2
Sport disciplines and risk of exercise-induced bronchoconstriction

Low-Risk Sports	Medium-Risk Sports	High-Risk Sports
All sports where the exercise lasts <5–8 min	Team sports where continuous exercise rarely lasts more than 5–8 min	All sports where the exercise lasts >5–8 min and/or is performed in special environments (ie, dry/cold air, chlorinated pools)
Track and field:	Soccer	Track and field:
• Sprint (100, 200, and 400 m)	Rugby	• Long distance (5000 and 10,000 m)
• Middle distance (800 and 1500 m)	American football	• 3000 m steeplechase
• Hurdles (100, 110, 400 m)	Basketball	• Walks (20 and 50 km)
• Jumps	Volleyball	• Marathon
• Throws	Handball	Cycling
Tennis	Baseball	Cross-country skiing
Fencing	Cricket	Downhill skiing
Gymnastics	Field hockey	Ice hockey
Boxing		Ice skating
Golf		High-altitude sports
Weightlifting		Triathlon
Body building		Pentathlon
Martial arts		Swimming
		Water polo

Carlsen and colleagues[47] first reported that the exercise load was related to the degree of bronchial hyperreactivity in both asthmatic and healthy swimmers. Some years later, the same investigators showed that the maximum decrease in forced expiratory volume at 1 second (FEV_1) after a treadmill test performed at 85% of maximal predicted heart rate (220, age) was significantly lower than the one recorded following a challenge at 95% (8.84% vs 25.11%; $P<.001$). Furthermore, although only 9 subjects (40%) fell $\geq$10% in FEV_1 after an exercise load at 85%, all the 20 subjects (100%) developed EIB after a 95% exercise test.[48]

Moreover, the longitudinal changes in the methacholine concentration needed to determine a 10% FEV_1 decrease in cross-country skiers were negatively correlated with the changes in the volume of physical activity only at an intensity level greater than 90% of maximal heart rate.[49] In addition, Stensrud and colleagues[50] observed increased airway reactivity to methacholine in elite athletes with increasing age and training volume.

Asthma is then most commonly found in athletes performing endurance activities, such as long-distance running, cycling, triathlon, and pentathlon. For example, in the study of Robson-Ansley and colleagues,[51] 32% of 208 runners from the 2010 London Marathon had asthma according to the validated Allergy Questionnaire for Athletes.[21] The high prevalence of EIB among endurance athletes has been mainly attributed to an increased minute ventilation through the mouth (bypassing the nasal filter) and exposure to allergens and pollutants.[52,53] In major national and international competitions, local pollen counts and forecasts (ie, www.polleninfo.org) should be therefore always made available in advance to athletes, their coaches, and medical teams.

Environmental factors also play a relevant role for athletes practicing winter sports. More than 1 out of 2 (54.8%) Swedish cross-country skiers were shown to have EIB in the study of Larsson and colleagues.[54] Similarly, the prevalence of bronchial hyperresponsiveness and clinical d asthma was 42% and 43%, respectively, in the 53 Swedish cross-country skiers studied by Sue-Chu and colleagues.[55] Such a high prevalence of asthma and EIB reported among Nordic and ice rink athletes has been attributed to the high ventilation of cold dry air during training and competition, in combination with the elevated emission of pollutants from fossil-fuelled ice resurfacing machines.[56,57]

Swimming has been long considered a safe and recommended sport activity for subjects with asthma because of the inhalation of humid air[58]; however, despite conflicting data,[59] an increased risk of EIB with swimming and pool attendance has been reported.[60,61] Furthermore, an association was shown between the number of chlorinated pools in the country and the prevalence of childhood asthma, independently from environmental conditions and subjects' socioeconomic status.[62] Bernard and colleagues[63] also reported that asthma development during adolescents was clearly associated with cumulative pool attendance before the age of 7. Competitive swimmers show a high prevalence of asthma and EIB,[64–66] with increased levels of leukotriene B4, a mixed eosinophilic-neutrophilic airways inflammation and evidence of bronchial epithelial damage.[63,67] These findings are thought to be the result of repeated hyperventilation challenges together with the exposure to chlorine-based derivatives, commonly used to disinfect swimming pools, such as trichloramine. This hypothesis is further supported by studies on occupational asthma in swimming pool workers and lifeguards[68] and by studies comparing exposures to non–chlorinated pools (copper-silver pools) versus chlorinated pools.[69]

At last, it is of interest to report that when the risk factors "type of sport" and "atopy" are combined in a logistic regression model, the relative risk of asthma is considerably high: 25-fold in atopic speed and power athletes, 42-fold in atopic long-distance runners, and 97-fold in atopic swimmers compared with nonatopic control subjects.[70]

SUMMARY

Although regular physical activity is strongly recommended for a proper prevention and management of chronic diseases, including asthma, evidence has been accumulating that intense and repeated exercise is associated with a higher prevalence of EIB both with and without underlying clinical asthma. EIB has been reported to be particularly frequent in swimming, endurance, and winter sports. Furthermore, in athletes, EIB seems to be only partly reversible, representing exercise itself as a causative factor of airway inflammation and symptoms. However, it is reassuring that, when properly diagnosed and optimally treated,[71] athletes with EIB are able to participate on the highest level with their peers with even more chances to succeed and win medals than others in the Olympic Games and other major international competitions.[72]

REFERENCES

1. Latimer-Cheung AE, Toll BA, Salovey P. Promoting increased physical activity and reduced inactivity. Lancet 2013;381(9861):114.
2. Moreira A, Bonini M, Pawankar R, et al. A World Allergy Organization international survey on physical activity as a treatment option for asthma and allergies. World Allergy Organ J 2014;7(1):34.
3. Moreira A, Delgado L, Haahtela T, et al. Physical training does not increase allergic inflammation in asthmatic children. Eur Respir J 2008;32(6):1570–5.
4. Eichenberger PA, Diener SN, Kofmehl R, et al. Effects of exercise training on airway hyperreactivity in asthma: a systematic review and meta-analysis. Sports Med 2013;43:1157–70.
5. Del Giacco SR, Garcia-Larsen V. Aerobic exercise training reduces bronchial hyper-responsiveness and serum pro-inflammatory cytokines in patients with asthma. Evid Based Med 2016;21(2):70.
6. Parsons JP, Hallstrand TS, Mastronarde JG, et al. An official American Thoracic Society clinical practice guideline: exercise-induced bronchoconstriction. Am J Respir Crit Care Med 2013;187(9):1016.
7. Walsh NP, Gleeson M, Shephard RJ, et al. Position statement. Part one: immune function and exercise. Exerc Immunol Rev 2011;17:6.
8. Lakier Smith L. Overtraining, excessive exercise, and altered immunity: is this a T helper-1 versus T helper-2 lymphocyte response? Sports Med 2003;33(5):347.
9. Del Giacco SR, Firinu D, Bjermer L, et al. Exercise and asthma: an overview. Eur Clin Respir J 2015;2:27984.
10. Jones KS, Buston MH, Wharton MJ. The effect of exercise on ventilator function in the child with asthma. Br J Dis Chest 1962;56:78–86.
11. Bonini M, Palange P. Exercise-induced bronchoconstriction: new evidence in pathogenesis, diagnosis and treatment. Asthma Res Pract 2015;1:2.
12. Godfrey S. Exercise-induced asthma. In: Clark TJH, Godfrey S, editors. Asthma. London: Chapman and Hall; 1977. p. 57–8.
13. Wenzel SE. Asthma: defining the persistent asthma phenotypes. Lancet 2006; 368:804–13.
14. Global INitiative on Asthma. Available at: http://ginasthma.org/. Accessed April 28, 2017.
15. Bonini S. EIB or not EIB? That is the question. Med Sci Sports Exerc 2008;40(9): 1565–6.

16. Weiler JM, Anderson SD, Randolph C, et al. Pathogenesis, prevalence, diagnosis, and management of exercise-induced bronchoconstriction: a practice parameter. Ann Allergy Asthma Immunol 2010;105:S1–47.
17. Smoliga JM, Weiss P, Rundell KW. Exercise induced bronchoconstriction in adults: evidence based diagnosis and management. BMJ 2016;352:h6951.
18. Anderson SD, Daviskas E. The mechanism of exercise-induced asthma is .... J Allergy Clin Immunol 2000;106:453–9.
19. McFadden ER. Hypothesis: exercise-induced asthma as a vascular phenomenon. Lancet 1990;1:880–3.
20. Price OJ, Hull JH, Ansley L, et al. Exercise-induced bronchoconstriction in athletes - a qualitative assessment of symptom perception. Respir Med 2016;120: 36–43.
21. Bonini M, Braido F, Baiardini I, et al. AQUA: allergy questionnaire for athletes. Development and validation. Med Sci Sports Exerc 2009;41(5):1034–41.
22. Ansley L, Kippelen P, Dickinson J, et al. Misdiagnosis of exercise-induced bronchoconstriction in professional soccer players. Allergy 2012;67(3):390–5.
23. Bonini M, Lapucci G, Petrelli G, et al. Predictive value of allergy and pulmonary function tests for the diagnosis of asthma in elite athletes. Allergy 2007;62(10): 1166–70.
24. Hull JH, Ansley L, Price OJ, et al. Eucapnic voluntary hyperpnea: gold standard for diagnosing exercise-induced bronchoconstriction in athletes? Sports Med 2016;46(8):1083–93.
25. Ansley L, Bonini M, Delgado L, et al. Pathophysiological mechanisms of exercise-induced anaphylaxis: an EAACI position statement. Allergy 2015;70(10): 1212–21.
26. Nielsen EW, Hull JH, Backer V. High prevalence of exercise-induced laryngeal obstruction in athletes. Med Sci Sports Exerc 2013;45(11):2030–5.
27. Bonini M, Di Mambro C, Calderon MA, et al. Beta-2 agonists for exercise-induced asthma. Cochrane Database Syst Rev 2013;(10):CD003564.
28. Bonini M, Permaul P, Kulkarni T, et al. Loss of salmeterol bronchoprotection against exercise in relation to ADRB2 Arg16Gly polymorphism and exhaled nitric oxide. Am J Respir Crit Care Med 2013;188(12):1407–12.
29. Salpeter SR, Buckley NS, Ormiston TM, et al. Meta-analysis: effect of long-acting beta-agonists on severe asthma exacerbations and asthma-related deaths. Ann Intern Med 2006;144(12):904–12.
30. The world anti-doping agency. Available at: www.wada-ama.org/. Accessed April 28, 2017.
31. Carlsen KH, Anderson SD, Bjermer L, et al. Exercise-induced asthma, respiratory and allergic disorders in elite athletes: epidemiology, mechanisms and diagnosis: part I of the report from the Joint Task Force of the European Respiratory Society (ERS) and the European Academy of Allergy and Clinical Immunology (EAACI) in cooperation with GA2LEN. Allergy 2008;63(4):387–403.
32. Randolph C. Exercise-induced bronchospasm in children. Clin Rev Allergy Immunol 2008;34(2):205–16.
33. Ventura MT, Cannone A, Sinesi D, et al. Sensitization, asthma and allergic disease in young soccer players. Allergy 2009;64(4):556–9.
34. Bousquet J, Van Cauwenberge P, Khaltaev N, Aria Workshop Group, World Health Organization. Allergic rhinitis and its impact on asthma. J Allergy Clin Immunol 2001;108(5 Suppl):S147–334.
35. Sandrock CE, Norris A. Infection in severe asthma exacerbations and critical asthma syndrome. Clin Rev Allergy Immunol 2015;48(1):104–13.

36. Voy RO. The US Olympic Committee experience with exercise-induced broncho-spasm, 1984. Med Sci Sports Exerc 1986;18:328–30.
37. Weiler JM, Layton T, Hunt M. Asthma in United States Olympic athletes who participated in the 1996 summer games. J Allergy Clin Immunol 1998;102:722–6.
38. Katelaris CH, Carrozzi FM, Burke TV, et al. A springtime olympics demands special consideration for allergic athletes. J Allergy Clin Immunol 2000;106:260–6.
39. Pignataro FS, Bonini M, Forgione A, et al. Asthma and gender: the female lung. Pharmacol Res 2017;119:384–90.
40. Romberg K, Tufvesson E, Bjermer L. Sex differences in asthma in swimmers and tennis players. Ann Allergy Asthma Immunol 2017;118(3):311–7.
41. Norqvist J, Eriksson L, Söderström L, et al. Self-reported physician-diagnosed asthma among Swedish adolescent, adult and former elite endurance athletes. J Asthma 2015;52(10):1046–53.
42. Settipane RJ, Hagy GW, Settipane GA. Long-term risk factors for developing asthma and allergic rhinitis: a 23-year follow-up study of college students. Allergy Proc 1994;15:21–5.
43. Braman SS, Barrows AA, De Cotiis BA, et al. Airway hyperresponsiveness in allergic rhinitis: a risk factor for asthma. Chest 1987;91:671–4.
44. Silvers WS, Poole JA. Exercise-induced rhinitis: a common disorder that adversely affects allergic and non-allergic athletes. Ann Allergy Asthma Immunol 2006;96(2):334–40.
45. Bonini S, Bonini M, Bousquet J, et al. Rhinitis and asthma in athletes: an ARIA document in collaboration with GA2LEN. Allergy 2006;61(6):681–92.
46. Helenius IJ, Rytilä P, Sarna S, et al. Effect of continuing or finishing high-level sports on airway inflammation, bronchial hyperresponsiveness, and asthma: a 5-year prospective follow-up study of 42 highly trained swimmers. J Allergy Clin Immunol 2002;109:962 8.
47. Carlsen KH, Oseid S, Odden H, et al. The response to heavy swimming exercise in children with and without bronchial asthma. In: Morehouse CA, editor. Children and exercise XIII. Champaign (IL): Human Kinetics Publishers, Inc; 1989. p. 351–60.
48. Carlsen KH, Engh G, Mørk M. Exercise-induced bronchoconstriction depends on exercise load. Respir Med 2000;94(8):750–5.
49. Heir T, Larsen S. The influence of training intensity, airway infections and environmental conditions on seasonal variations in bronchial responsiveness in cross-country skiers. Scand J Med Sci Sports 1995;5:152–9.
50. Stensrud T, Mykland KV, Gabrielsen K, et al. Bronchial hyperresponsiveness in skiers: field test versus methacholine provocation? Med Sci Sports Exerc 2007; 39:1681–6.
51. Robson-Ansley P, Howatson G, Tallent J, et al. Prevalence of allergy and upper respiratory tract symptoms in runners of the London marathon. Med Sci Sports Exerc 2012;44(6):999–1004.
52. Helenius I, Haahtela T. Allergy and asthma in elite summer sport athletes. J Allergy Clin Immunol 2000;106:444–52.
53. McCreanor J, Cullinan P, Nieuwenhuijsen MJ, et al. Respiratory effects of exposure to diesel traffic in persons with asthma. N Engl J Med 2007;357:2348–58.
54. Larsson K, Ohlsén P, Larsson L, et al. High prevalence of asthma in cross country skiers. BMJ 1993;307(6915):1326–9.
55. Sue-Chu M, Larsson L, Bjermer L. Prevalence of asthma in young cross-country skiers in central Scandinavia: differences between Norway and Sweden. Respir Med 1996;90(2):99–105.

56. Sue-Chu M, Henriksen AH, Bjermer L. Non-invasive evaluation of lower airway inflammation in hyper-responsive elite cross-country skiers and asthmatics. Respir Med 1999;93:719–25.
57. Rundell KW. High levels of airborne ultrafine and fine particulate matter in indoor ice arenas. Inhal Toxicol 2003;15:237–50.
58. Goodman M, Hays S. Asthma and swimming: a meta-analysis. J Asthma 2008; 45:639–47.
59. Valeriani F, Protano C, Vitali M, et al. Swimming attendance during childhood and development of asthma: meta-analysis. Pediatr Int 2017;59(5):614–21.
60. Bernard A, Carbonnelle S, de Burbure C, et al. Chlorinated pool attendance, atopy, and the risk of asthma during childhood. Environ Health Perspect 2006; 114:1567–73.
61. Andersson M, Hedman L, Nordberg G, et al. Swimming pool attendance is related to asthma among atopic school children: a population-based study. Environ Health 2015;14:37.
62. Nickmilder M, Bernard A. Ecological association between childhood asthma and availability of indoor chlorinated swimming pools in Europe. Occup Environ Med 2007;64:37–46.
63. Bernard A, Nickmilder M, Dumont X. Chlorinated pool attendance, airway epithelium defects and the risks of allergic diseases in adolescents: interrelationships revealed by circulating biomarkers. Environ Res 2015;140:119–26.
64. Fisk MZ, Steigerwald MD, Smoliga JM, et al. Asthma in swimmers: a review of the current literature. Phys Sportsmed 2010;38(4):28–34.
65. Stadelmann K, Stensrud T, Carlsen KH. Respiratory symptoms and bronchial responsiveness in competitive swimmers. Med Sci Sports Exerc 2011;43:375–81.
66. Mountjoy M, Fitch K, Boulet LP, et al. Prevalence and characteristics of asthma in the aquatic disciplines. J Allergy Clin Immunol 2015;136(3):588–94.
67. Moreira A, Delgado L, Palmares C, et al. Competitive swimmers with allergic asthma show a mixed type of airway inflammation. Eur Respir J 2008;31:1139–41.
68. Rosenman KD, Millerick-May M, Reilly MJ, et al. Swimming facilities and work-related asthma. J Asthma 2015;52(1):52–8.
69. Bernard A, Nickmilder M, Voisin C, et al. Impact of chlorinated swimming pool attendance on the respiratory health of adolescents. Pediatrics 2009;124:1110–8.
70. Helenius IJ, Tikkanen HO, Sarna S, et al. Asthma and increased bronchial responsiveness in elite athletes: atopy and sport event as risk factors. J Allergy Clin Immunol 1998;101:646–52.
71. Bonini M, Bachert C, Baena-Cagnani CE, et al, ARIA Initiative, in collaboration with the WHO Collaborating Center for Asthma, Rhinitis. What we should learn from the London Olympics. Curr Opin Allergy Clin Immunol 2013;13(1):1–3.
72. McKenzie DC, Fitch KD. The asthmatic athlete: inhaled beta-2 agonists, sport performance, and doping. Clin J Sport Med 2011;21(1):46–50.

Testing for Exercise-Induced Bronchoconstriction

John D. Brannan, PhD[a],*, Celeste Porsbjerg, MD, PhD[b]

KEYWORDS

- Exercise-induced bronchoconstriction • Eucapnic voluntary hyperpnea • Mannitol
- Airway hyperresponsiveness

KEY POINTS

- Exercise-induced bronchoconstriction (EIB) is an indicator of active and treatable pathology in persons with asthma, but also can occur in persons who do not have a clinical diagnosis of asthma.
- The objective documentation of the presence and severity of EIB also permits the identification of an individual who may be at risk during a recreational sporting activity or when exercising as occupational duty.
- Laboratory exercise challenge testing can have limitations in the assessment of EIB, as the ambient air conditions cannot often be well controlled, preventing an optimal airway dehydrating stimulus to induce EIB.
- Surrogate challenge tests, such as eucapnic voluntary hyperpnea and the osmotic challenge tests (eg, inhaled mannitol), have considerable practical advantages over laboratory exercise testing.

INTRODUCTION

Exercise-induced bronchoconstriction (EIB) is the term used to describe the transient narrowing of the airways that occurs during, although most commonly following vigorous exercise.[1] EIB is the term used to describe airway narrowing to exercise in both those with clinical symptoms of asthma (in the past termed "exercise-induced asthma") and those who experience EIB in the absence of clinical asthma.[2] Although the initial aims of developing protocols for exercise testing were to identify airway hyperresponsiveness (AHR) in those with active

---

Disclosure Statement: Dr J.D. Brannan was involved in the development of inhaled mannitol (Aridol/Osmohale). He receives a 10% portion of the royalties from his prior employer, Royal Prince Alfred Hospital, that are paid by the manufacturer, Pharmaxis Ltd, Australia. He holds shares in Pharmaxis Ltd that he purchased himself. Dr C. Porsbjerg has no conflict of interest.
[a] Department of Respiratory and Sleep Medicine, John Hunter Hospital, Lookout Road, New Lambton, New South Wales 2305, Australia; [b] Respiratory Research Unit, Department of Respiratory Medicine, Bispebjerg Hospital, Bispebjerg Bakke 23, Copenhagen 2400, Denmark
* Corresponding author.
E-mail address: john.brannan@health.nsw.gov.au

asthma, testing also is used for the identification of EIB in recreational or competitive athletes.[1] These tests also have found a place in screening subjects susceptible to EIB who may be at risk from vigorous exercise during a recreational activity (eg, SCUBA diving) or an occupational duty (eg, defense, rescue, and police recruits).[3–5] A variety of protocols for exercise testing have been established, such as treadmill running or cycling on an ergometer in adults.[1,6] Protocols in children using treadmill or shuttle running, as well as a jumping castle, have been used.[7–9]

Given that exercise per se was not required to cause EIB and that there are practical difficulties with exercise, the development of surrogate tests have made testing for EIB more clinically accessible and standardizable. The development of the bronchial provocation tests (BPTs), eucapnic voluntary hyperpnea (EVH), and the osmotic challenge tests (eg, hypertonic saline, inhaled dry powder mannitol), have found a place to identify both the presence and severity of EIB[10,11] (Fig. 1). Documenting EIB identifies an individual who is highly likely to benefit from pharmacologic treatments and strategies (eg, warm-up exercise) to inhibit EIB.[1]

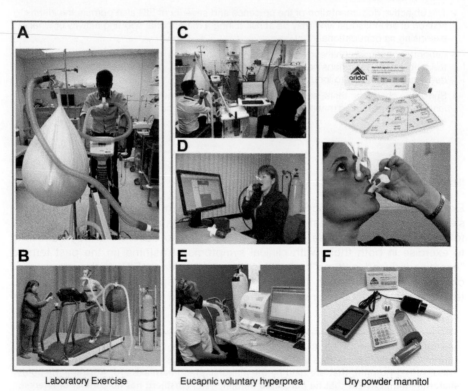

Laboratory Exercise   Eucapnic voluntary hyperpnea   Dry powder mannitol

Fig. 1. An example of equipment required to perform laboratory exercise, eucapnic voluntary hyperpnea, or inhaled mannitol challenge testing. Exercise challenge testing: (A) Cycling exercise using a cycle ergometer. (B) Running exercise using a treadmill. Eucapnic voluntary hyperpnea: (C) Noncommercial system using sourced equipment. (D) Commercial device known as the hyperventilometer. (E) Commercial device known as the EucapSys system. (F) Mannitol challenge test kit and supporting equipment. (Courtesy of [A, C] ergoline GmbH, Bitz, Germany; [E] SMTEC SA, Nyon, Switzerland; and [F] Pharmaxis Ltd, Frenchs Forest, New South Wales, Australia.)

MECHANISMS OF BRONCHIAL PROVOCATION TESTS TO IDENTIFY EXERCISE-INDUCED BRONCHOCONSTRICTION
Indirect Bronchial Provocation Tests

Indirect BPTs include tests that require dry air hyperpnea (eg, exercise, EVH) or osmotic aerosols (eg, mannitol). These tests share a common primary stimulus for inducing airway narrowing, which is the increase in the osmolarity of the airway surface liquid[12] (**Fig. 2**). With exercise or EVH, the increase in osmolarity is a result of evaporative water loss. The osmotic aerosols raise the airway osmolarity directly, for example, by the inhalation of the osmotic agent. The osmotic stimulus causes the release of mediators of bronchoconstriction including histamine, prostaglandins, leukotrienes, and neurokinins, from inflammatory cells (mast cells, eosinophils).[13–15] These mediators then act on the airway smooth muscle directly or indirectly via the sensory nerves to cause contraction and the airways to narrow. (See the article by Pascale Kippelen and colleagues, "Mechanisms and Biomarkers of Exercise-Induced Bronchoconstriction," elsewhere in this issue). The key pathophysiological features that lead to EIB are the presence of airway inflammation and the hyperresponsive airway smooth muscle.[1]

It is now understood that mediator release can occur to some degree in those with no airway responses to indirect stimuli, suggesting that smooth muscle sensitivity is essential.[14,16] There is good association between the severity of the airway response to exercise, EVH, and mannitol, in both individuals with asthma and elite athletes[17,18] (**Figs. 3** and **4**). Another common feature with indirect stimuli is a refractory period following repeat stimulus within a short time period. It is well established that

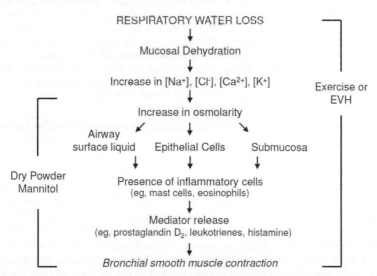

Fig. 2. A schematic outlining the key events that result in AHR due to hyperpnea with dry air in persons with asthma that occurs during or following vigorous exercise or a EVH challenge. The osmotic challenge test inhaled dry powder mannitol mimics the effects of dry air hyperpnea by increasing the osmolarity of the airway surface. For all these stimuli, an important feature is the presence of airway inflammation in association with a sensitive airway smooth muscle. (*Adapted from* Porsbjerg C, Brannan JD. Alternatives to exercise challenge for the objective assessment of exercise-induced bronchospasm: eucapnic voluntary hyperpnoea and the osmotic challenge tests. Breathe 2010;7(1):60; Reproduced with permission from the © ERS 2010. Breathe Sep 2010, 7(1):52–63; DOI: 10.1183/18106838.0701.053.)

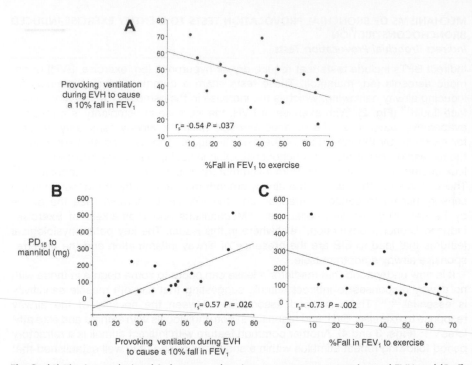

Fig. 3. (A) The interrelationship between the airway response to exercise and EVH and (B, C) when both are compared with mannitol in the same 15 asthmatic subjects. The airway response to exercise is expressed as a % fall in FEV_1; the airway response to EVH is expressed as the provoking ventilation to induce a 10% fall in FEV_1 (obtained during a multistage EVH challenge test) and the airway response to mannitol expressed as the cumulative dose to cause a 15% fall in FEV_1 (PD_{15}). (*Data from* Brannan JD, Koskela H, Anderson SD, et al. Responsiveness to mannitol in asthmatic subjects with exercise- and hyperventilation-induced asthma. Am J Respir Crit Care Med 1998;158(4):1120–6.)

50% of subjects with EIB can have a 50% inhibition to a second exercise test within 4 hours of the initial test.[19]

Direct Bronchial Provocation Tests

Direct tests use single agonists administered via inhalation (histamine, or more commonly methacholine)[20] that cause airway narrowing by acting on specific airway receptors on bronchial smooth muscle to cause contraction and airway narrowing. It is appreciated that AHR to direct BPTs may cause bronchoconstriction for reasons other than airway inflammation, such as airway remodeling and reductions in airway caliber.[21] Epidemiology studies comparing direct and indirect tests to assess EIB in children initially revealed limitations in using direct tests, as they did not identify EIB in some subjects.[8,22] It is now clear direct tests do not predict presence of EIB in adults suspected of asthma.[23,24] This may in part be explained by both methacholine and histamine being less potent bronchoconstricting stimuli when compared with either prostaglandins and leukotrienes, which are implicated in EIB.[25]

More recent findings demonstrate in persons suspected of asthma who were given a clinical diagnosis based on results from an exercise challenge that up to 50% had no AHR to methacholine.[23] Thus, no AHR to direct stimuli can be common in both EIB alone and in newly diagnosed asthma with EIB. The increasing studies reporting failure

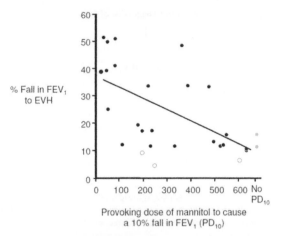

Fig. 4. In elite athletes, the relationship of the airway response to EVH expressed as a % fall in FEV_1 and the airway response to mannitol expressed as the cumulative dose to cause a 10% fall in FEV_1 (PD_{10}). Most who responded to both tests (*black dots*) with those positive to EVH alone (*gray dots*) and those responsive to mannitol alone (*white dots*). In 24 subjects who had airway responses to both tests, there was a good relationship between % fall in FEV_1 to EVH and the PD_{10} to mannitol (r_p = 0.61, r_s = 0.70, P<.01). (*Data from* Holzer K, Anderson SD, Chan HK, et al. Mannitol as a challenge test to identify exercise-induced bronchoconstriction in elite athletes. Am J Respir Crit Care Med 2003;167(4):534–7.)

of direct tests to identify EIB has led current guidelines to not recommend the use of direct BPTs for the diagnosis of EIB.[1]

BRONCHIAL PROVOCATION TESTS FOR EXERCISE-INDUCED BRONCHOCONSTRICTION: COMMON FEATURES AND CONSIDERATIONS

BPTs are clinically useful to identify AHR in persons with normal to near-normal lung function who have symptoms suggestive of asthma or EIB (**Fig. 5**). It can be clinically unnecessary and unsafe to perform these tests in these subjects with abnormal lung function identified with a forced expiratory volume in 1 second (FEV_1) less than 70% of predicted normal. If reversibility to a standard dose of bronchodilator is documented in these patients, it would be suspected that the presence of AHR is likely and the likelihood of EIB will be high. For subjects with abnormal spirometry and no beta$_2$ agonist reversibility, a full respiratory workup, including gas transfer and plethysmographic lung volumes, would be warranted.[1]

The purpose of any BPT is to provide a stimulus that is in keeping with the real-life stimuli that has produced the patients' symptoms. Further, the stimulus should be administered in a safe and controlled manner to document an abnormal change in airway caliber. The preferred measurement to document this change is the FEV_1 measured with spirometry. The cutoff values to demonstrate an abnormal response (% fall in FEV_1) have been determined by the mean and 2 SDs observed in nonasthmatic subjects without EIB[11] (see **Fig. 5**).

The rate of change of airway osmolarity is considered an important feature of achieving an optimal bronchoconstricting stimulus to exercise, EVH, and mannitol. If the stimulus causes a slow osmotic change to the airway surface from a prolonged test performed outside the test recommendations, the potency of the stimulus is diminished.[26]

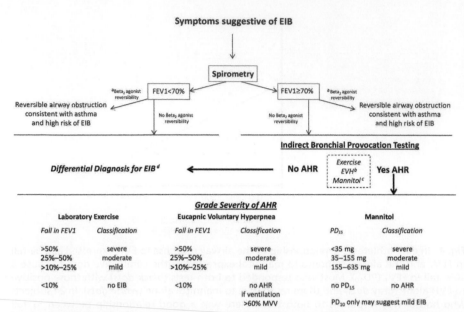

Symptoms suggestive of EIB

Spirometry

| Reversible airway obstruction consistent with asthma and high risk of EIB | ᵃBeta₂ agonist reversibility | FEV1<70% | | FEV1≥70% | ᵃBeta₂ agonist reversibility | Reversible airway obstruction consistent with asthma and high risk of EIB |

No Beta₂ agonist reversibility   No Beta₂ agonist reversibility

Indirect Bronchial Provocation Testing

Differential Diagnosis for EIB ᵈ ⟵ No AHR | Exercise EVHᵇ Mannitolᶜ | **Yes AHR**

Grade Severity of AHR

Laboratory Exercise		Eucapnic Voluntary Hyperpnea		Mannitol	
Fall in FEV1	*Classification*	*Fall in FEV1*	*Classification*	*PD₁₅*	*Classification*
>50%	severe	>50%	severe	<35 mg	severe
25%–50%	moderate	25%–50%	moderate	35–155 mg	moderate
>10%–25%	mild	>10%–25%	mild	155–635 mg	mild
<10%	no EIB	<10%	no AHR if ventilation >60% MVV	no PD₁₅	no AHR
				PD₁₀ only may suggest mild EIB	

Fig. 5. An algorithm for the decision to perform an indirect bronchial provocation test in persons with symptoms suggestive of EIB, including the test options and test outcomes, which include the cutoff values for a positive test and the classification of the airway response to a grade severity of AHR. ᵃ Demonstrating reversibility in FEV₁ of 12% and 200 mL. ᵇ FEV₁ ≥75% for EVH challenge. ᶜ Subject to availability in the United States. ᵈ Very mild AHR may cause variable responses to all tests and if EIB is still strongly suspect, a repeat test may be warranted. (*Adapted from* Weiler JM, Brannan JD, Randolph CC, et al. Exercise-induced bronchoconstriction update-2016. J Allergy Clin Immunol 2016;138(5):1292–5.e36; with permission.)

The stimulus to elicit EIB can be delivered in 2 distinct forms[1] (**Fig. 6**):

1. Exercise or EVH: A bolus or "ungraded challenge," whereby the challenge delivers a single episode (or dose) of hyperpnea to cause an unspecified fall in FEV₁. The FEV₁ is measured before and regularly for at least 10 to 15 minutes following hyperpnea. The maximum fall in FEV₁ is expressed as a percentage of the baseline FEV₁ and is taken as the response. The severity of the response is classified by the final percentage fall in FEV₁, a measure of airway reactivity (see **Fig. 5**).

2. Mannitol: A dose-response or "graded challenge," whereby the agent is administered by inhaling increasing doses to cause a specified fall in FEV₁. This graded challenge permits the construction of a dose-response curve to determine the provoking dose (PD) to induce the specified fall, usually 15% (PD₁₅) or 10% (PD₁₀).[17,18] The PD₁₅ or PD₁₀ is a measure of sensitivity. An index of airway reactivity also can be documented by calculating the response-dose ratio, defined as the final % fall in FEV₁ divided by the cumulative dose of mannitol that caused that fall (% fall in FEV₁ per milligram of mannitol).

It should be recognized that medications for the treatment of asthma, caffeine-containing drinks, and physical exercise before testing can attenuate the airway response to all these challenge tests with similar potency.[27] For this reason, patients should be informed of the most appropriate times to withhold from these treatments, foods, or physical activity[1] (**Table 1**).

Baseline FEV$_1$ >70% of predicted

Bolus dose / ungraded challenge		Dose response / graded challenge
Exercise Calculate Predicted HR & MVV (if ventilation can be measured) Encourage subject to exercise 2–3 min to reach maximum intensity and sustain this level of intensity so total exercise time is no more than 8 min or 6 min in children On completion measure duplicate FEV$_1$ values at 5 min intervals for 20–30 min (FEV1 at 1 or 3 min post exercise optional) A positive test is recorded if a ≥10% fall in FEV$_1$ in adults and ≥15% fall in children	**EVH** Baseline FEV1 >75% recommended. Maximum voluntary ventilation (MVV) is calculated from baseline FEV$_1$ and is equal to MVV = 35 X FEV$_1$ Encourage subject to voluntarily hyperventilate to achieve at least or greater than 60% of MVV throughout 6 min On completion measure duplicate FEV$_1$ values at 1, 3, 5, 10, 15, & 20 min A positive test occurs if a ≥10% fall at two time points is achieved after the test	**Mannitol** Calculate 15% fall from baseline Subject inhales a 0 mg capsule. 60 s later FEV$_1$ is measured in duplicate, baseline FEV$_1$ recorded Separate doses of 5, 10, 20, 40, 80 (2 x 40), 160 (4 x 40), 160 & 160 mg are administered. 60 s after each dose FEV$_1$ measured in duplicate A fall ≥15% in FEV$_1$ from baseline or an incremental (between dose) fall of 10% at a cumulative dose ≤645 mg is a positive test

Administer beta$_2$ agonist

Post bronchodilator FEV$_1$

Fig. 6. A brief comparison of the fundamental similarities and differences in the protocols required to perform laboratory exercise, EVH, and mannitol challenge testing. (*Adapted from* Porsbjerg C, Brannan JD. Alternatives to exercise challenge for the objective assessment of exercise induced bronchospasm: eucapnic voluntary hyperpnoea and the osmotic challenge tests. Breathe 2010; 7(1):60; Reproduced with permission from the ©ERS 2010. Breathe Sep 2010, 7(1):52–63; DOI: 10.1183/18106838.0701.053.)

All challenge testing should be conducted by trained personnel using standardized protocols. Reproducible full spirometry in accordance with American Thoracic Society/European Respiratory Society standards should be performed at baseline (documenting at least FEV$_1$ and forced vital capacity) before the challenge stimulus. Full spirometry is not performed during or after the challenge to prevent patient fatigue. A common feature with all indirect challenge tests is the best FEV$_1$ at each time point following exercise or EVH, or 60 seconds following each administered dose of mannitol, is used for the calculation of % fall from baseline FEV$_1$. Once the maximum % fall in FEV$_1$ following exercise or EVH has been established, or on the documentation of the desired 15% fall during a mannitol challenge, bronchodilator is administered. Spirometry is then repeated 10 minutes following bronchodilator and the FEV$_1$ post bronchodilator should be within 5% of the pretest baseline FEV$_1$ (see **Fig. 6**).

Significant falls in FEV$_1$ are more common with exercise and EVH and this cannot necessarily be predicted by the subjects' baseline FEV$_1$. In patients with known EIB and a concomitant history of asthma requiring treatment, large falls in FEV$_1$ may be expected with exercise and EVH, and in these subjects a dose-response challenge has been recommended as preferable.[1] Laboratories are required to have available a bronchodilator (rapidly acting beta$_2$ agonist in a pressurized metered dose inhaler) with the option of nebulized bronchodilator with a supply of oxygen for severe falls in FEV$_1$.

Table 1
The recommended withdrawal times for medications, foods, and physical activity before performing challenge testing with exercise, eucapnic voluntary hyperpnea, or inhaled mannitol

Medication/Activity/Food	Recommended Time to Withhold Before Challenge Testing
Short-acting beta$_2$ agonist (albuterol, terbutaline)	8 h
Long-acting beta$_2$ agonist (salmeterol, eformoterol)	24 h
Long-acting beta$_2$ agonist in combination with an inhaled corticosteroid (salmeterol/fluticasone, formoterol/budesonide)	24 h
Ultra-long-acting beta$_2$ agonists (indacaterol, olodaterol, vilanterol)	$\geq$72 h
Inhaled corticosteroid (budesonide, fluticasone propionate, beclomethasone)	6 h
Long-acting inhaled corticosteroid (fluticasone furoate)	24 h
Leukotriene receptor antagonists (montelukast, zafirlukast)	4 d
Leukotriene synthesis inhibitors (zileuton/slow-release zileuton)	12 h/16 h
Antihistamines (loratadine, cetirizine, fexofenadine)	72 h
Short-acting muscarinic acetylcholine antagonist (ipratropium bromide)	12 h
Long-acting muscarinic acetylcholine antagonist (tiotropium bromide, aclidinium bromide, glycopyrronium)	$\geq$72 h
Cromones (sodium cromoglycate, nedocromil sodium)	4 h
Xanthines (theophylline)	24 h
Caffeine	24 h
Vigorous exercise	>4 h

Adapted from Weiler JM, Brannan JD, Randolph CC, et al. Exercise-induced bronchoconstriction update-2016. J Allergy Clin Immunol 2016;138(5):1292–5.e36; with permission.

There is no single test that can identify all individuals who have EIB. There can be variations in the airway response with exercise compared with EVH and mannitol, as well as evidence of variation with the same test in an individual.[18,23,28,29] It has been reported that the response to exercise on an initial challenge only has a 62% sensitivity of predicting EIB on repeat challenge.[23,28] This lack of reproducibility has generally been observed predominately in persons with milder AHR, although not in all cases.[28] If EIB is still strongly suspected, a second test may be required or a test using a stronger stimuli (eg, EVH) may be warranted for confirmation[1] (see **Fig. 5**). EVH is considered more potent compared with exercise and can identify AHR more frequently.[30–32] Mannitol also has been shown to identify AHR 1.4 times more than a 10% fall in FEV_1 to exercise and 1.65 times more if a 15% fall to exercise is considered as an abnormal response.[23]

Common symptoms that result from airway narrowing to BPTs are the common symptoms associated with asthma, such as wheeze, chest tightness, and cough. Although these symptoms may be directly the result of bronchospasm, coughing also may result from indirect tests due to the osmotic activation of airway sensory nerves.[33] Coughing during a mannitol challenge test is common; however, the severity of cough can be broad, and its prevalence has been well characterized in Phase 3 studies.[23,34] These studies in large populations have demonstrated that very few challenge tests (1%–2%) are stopped prematurely due to excessive cough. Cough when inhaling mannitol can occur independently of bronchoconstriction.[35]

Mannitol-provoked cough is significantly less in individuals without asthma compared with those with asthma, and the cough is reduced following treatment with an inhaled corticosteroid in asthma, suggesting an inflammatory component to the osmotically induced cough response.[35] Mannitol-provoked cough is thought to excite the same sensory nerves as hypertonic saline and dry air hyperpnea.[33] However, the heightened cough sensitivity in individuals with asthma also may involve activation of mechanoreceptors during bronchospasm.[35]

LABORATORY EXERCISE PROVOCATION

Exercise-testing protocols using treadmill were initially developed in the 1970s to identify EIB in children. This led to the eventual development of protocols for use in adults, which included both running using a treadmill and then cycling with a cycle ergometer[12] (see **Fig. 1**A, B).

Laboratory protocols for exercise are well defined and have been updated in current guidelines,[1,36] understanding that the osmotic and thermal effects of respiratory water loss are key to identifying EIB and care should be taken when testing to achieve a maximal dehydrating stimulus to the airways. Initially the exercise intensity needs to be increased rapidly, preferably in the first 2-minutes of exercise. This can be observed by demonstrating a heart rate of at least 85% in adults and 95% in children.[1] Testing should continue for an additional 4 to 6 minutes at this peak intensity, delivering no more than 8 minutes of exercise in total for adults, 6 minutes for children.

To ensure that the optimal dehydrating stimulus is provided, the real-time recording of the minute ventilation, as well as making sure exercise is performed with the subject inhaling air with the lowest possible water content. The latter can be delivered directly to the subject from a tank of compressed air using a demand valve that delivers high flow rates to a 2-way non-rebreathing valve mouth piece, or indirectly via a reservoir (eg, Douglas bag) (see **Fig. 1**A, B). The maximum voluntary ventilation (MVV) a subject can achieve is calculated by multiplying the baseline $FEV_1 \times 35$. The minimum level of ventilation reached and sustained during the exercise challenge should be at least 60% of MVV, or at least $21 \times FEV_1$. Elite athletes may achieve this level of ventilation early in the exercise test and higher levels of ventilation will be required, in turn requiring a greater exercise intensity for this group.

Following full spirometry before exercise, FEV_1 is performed after exercise and at 5-minute intervals for 20 to 30 minutes. For reasons of safety, it is recommended that FEV_1 measurements are made at 1 and 3 minutes after exercise if it is suspected that the patient has bronchoconstriction during exercise.[6] This may be identified indirectly by noting reductions in ventilation during exercise, which also may be associated with symptoms during exercise.

The high intensity of exercise required to identify EIB limits its usefulness in some children and adults, particularly the elderly or impaired (eg, obese). Exercise testing for children has recently been made more accessible and simpler using a jumping castle protocol; however, it requires a specially air-conditioned room.[9] Testing for EIB requires at least 2 trained personnel in attendance for up to an hour, adding significantly to the expense of the test. The equipment required to perform the exercise adequately (eg, treadmill or bicycle ergometer) can be expensive and space occupying, confining testing to a specialist laboratory.

The reproducibility of the %fall in FEV_1 to exercise has been well characterized in persons with known asthma as well as a large number of subjects with suspected asthma.[28,37] Although it may be more difficult to see consistent positive test results in persons with mild AHR to exercise, consistent positive tests are more often observed in patients with falls in FEV_1 greater than 20% (**Table 2**).

EUCAPNIC VOLUNTARY HYPERPNEA

EVH (eucapnic hyperventilation or also known as isocapnic hyperventilation) was developed from the understanding that the ventilation reached and sustained, and the water content of the air inspired were the most important determinants of EIB.[38] Thus, a patient can voluntarily hyperventilate a source of dry air containing 4.9% to 5.0% carbon dioxide to maintain eucapnia, with the remainder of the gas mixture containing 21% oxygen and the balance nitrogen.[39] The characteristics of the airway response to EVH are very similar to exercise; however, the patient's maximum level of ventilation can be reached more rapidly with voluntary hyperventilation, thus reducing the required time for the EVH test, when compared with the exercise challenge.

The equipment to perform an EVH challenge requires less space and equipment than exercise (see **Fig. 1C–E**). Noncommercial or home-made systems similar to those that were first developed are still in use[26] (see **Fig. 1C**). The required apparatus can be easily sourced and the initial setup is relatively inexpensive compared with exercise. Real-time measurement of ventilation is recommended, and a pre-prepared gas mixture is required, which adds to the cost of the test. This system requires a large meteorologic balloon as a gas reservoir and the balloon is filled with at least 90 L of the dry air mixture containing 5% CO_2. The patient inhales the air via a 2-way valve and is encouraged to hyperventilate sufficiently to keep the balloon at a constant volume, while the gas from the cylinder refills the balloon via a rotameter at the target ventilation. This system provides constant feedback to patients on their ventilation, while the investigator can encourage "deeper" or "faster" breathing if required. This mixture keeps end-tidal CO_2 levels within the normal or eucapnic range between 40 and 105 L/min in subjects with FEV_1 values greater than 1.5 L.[39] If a subject, such as an elite athlete, has a level of ventilation value beyond this range, then a mixing

Table 2
The reproducibility of the % fall in FEV_1 to 2 exercise tests separated by approximately 4 days in both adults and children with mild symptoms of asthma

Group	n	Highest %Fall FEV_1 Mean ± SD	%Fall FEV_1 95% Probability Interval	%Fall 2 Tests Mean	%Fall Difference SD
Total	373	11.0 ± 9.4	± 10.8	8.2	7.6
Adults	278	10.4 ± 8.9	± 9.7	7.9	6.9
Children	95	12.6 ± 10.5	± 13.4	9.3	9.5
Two tests ≥10% fall	72	24.7 ± 9.7	± 14.6	20.8	10.3
Two tests ≥15% fall	34	29.4 ± 8.5	± 12.2	25.9	8.6
Two tests ≥20% fall	19	34.0 ± 8.2	± 14.3	30.1	10.1
One test ≥10% fall	89	14.3 ± 4.8	± 15.7	9.4	11.1
Two tests <10% fall	212	4.9 ± 2.9	± 5.2	3.5	3.7
Two tests <15% fall	288	6.8 ± 4.2	± 7.1	4.9	5.0

Data from Anderson SD, Pearlman DS, Rundell KW, et al. Reproducibility of the airway response to an exercise protocol standardized for intensity, duration, and inspired air conditions, in subjects with symptoms suggestive of asthma. Respir Res 2010;11(1):120.

device can be used to adjust and monitor the CO_2 concentration to maintain eucapnia. It is important that eucapnia (38–42 mm Hg) is maintained during an EVH challenge, as hypocapnia has long been known as a stimulus for bronchoconstriction.[40]

There are now commercial systems that also require gas mixtures that use a demand valve directly attached to the source of gas, with incentive devices on computer screens to help the subject achieve the target ventilation (see **Fig. 1**D). Another commercial system permits the breath-by-breath delivery of dry air with the addition of CO_2[41] (see **Fig. 1**E). These systems may in the long-term be cheaper to run, as separate sources of dry air and CO_2 are cheaper than a pre-prepared gas mixture.

There are a number of different protocols for EVH; however, the most accepted standardized protocol uses the pre-prepared gas mixture inhaled at room temperature for 6 minutes.[1,36] The target ventilation is 30 × the baseline FEV_1 and it has been demonstrated that most subjects are able to achieve this target. The minimum level for a valid test may be set as low as 17.5 times the FEV_1 for 6 minutes to be consistent with exercise ventilation; however, if the minimum ventilation is not reached, the test may be invalid and need repeating. Cooling the air can reduce the time of the challenge; however, it is an expensive addition, and for most assessments is unnecessary. At the end of the period of ventilation, FEV_1 is measured in duplicate immediately after challenge and at 3, 5, 10, 15, and 20 minutes.

In susceptible patients, in particular those with known asthma, more severe falls in FEV_1 could be achieved with this 6-minute protocol, and it is for this reason these subjects are recommended to be excluded from performing EVH[1] (see **Fig. 5**). For known asthmatic individuals, a 4-minute protocol at 21 × the FEV_1 has been used, as well as a multistage protocol requiring 3-minute periods of ventilation at 10.5, 21.0, and 31.0 times FEV_1.[17,42] If using a multistage protocol in known asthmatic individuals, measurements of FEV_1 are made following each EVH stage at 1, 3, 5, and 7 minutes. If there is no further fall at 7 minutes, the subject proceeds to the next level of ventilation. Progressive protocols can induce refractoriness, which leads to an attenuated response at the next ventilation level in some patients. For this reason, progressive protocols should not be used routinely. AHR may occur during ventilation, and any sudden falls in ventilation rate could be an indication of bronchoconstriction. In such cases, the test may need to cease, and FEV_1 measured immediately.

A fall in FEV_1 ≥10% from the prechallenge value is defined as a positive test, and the severity of the fall in FEV_1 defines the severity of the AHR (see **Fig. 5**). It is recommended that the fall in FEV_1 should be sustained, with the subject having at least a 10% fall in FEV_1 recorded at 2 consecutive time points after the challenge.[1,36] A fall of 15% has been suggested for athletes in whom it was demonstrated a high likelihood of obtaining at least 2 consecutive falls greater than 10%.[43]

EVH has been observed to identify more cases of EIB than laboratory exercise tests, and it is as sensitive as field exercise testing for athletes.[30–32] This is likely due to the higher levels of ventilation that can be rapidly achieved and sustained using EVH compared with laboratory exercise on a bicycle or treadmill. Thus, persons with mild EIB with a negative response to an exercise protocol may have a positive response to the 6-minute dry air EVH protocol. EVH is now well established and is preferred for the diagnosis of EIB in elite athletes.[1,36] Assessments of the reproducibility of the airway response to EVH are limited to small populations of either athletes or nonathletes.[10,29,44,45] Variations around the diagnostic cutoff value of 10% with mild AHR occur, similar to the observed variations with exercise [Anderson 2010][28], suggesting the possible need for 2 tests in borderline responses if EIB is still suspected.[1,29] However, those with moderate falls in FEV_1 to EVH appear to have adequate reproducible airway responses over 3 and 6 weeks.[10,45]

MANNITOL BRONCHIAL PROVOCATION TEST

The mannitol challenge test is an osmotic challenge tests that is commercially available as a disposable test kit consisting of dry powder mannitol and a low-resistance dry powder inhaler (Aridol/Osmohale)[34] (see **Fig. 1F**). The test has been approved by regulatory authorities in Australia, United States, European Union, and Korea and is also available in some other regions.[46] At the time of writing, Aridol is available for use only in approved clinical trials in the United States; however, there are prospects for its reintroduction to the wider US market.

The mannitol challenge test was developed in an attempt to make an indirect BPT more clinically accessible so the test could move beyond the clinical laboratory to be performed safely in a clinical office setting. Before this osmotic challenge, testing was performed using aerosols of hypertonic saline generated by large-volume ultrasonic nebulizers that were confined to clinical laboratories.[11] There were additional disadvantages with nebulization, such as variation in the delivered dose of aerosol, hygienic problems related to the patient expiration of the wet aerosols and exposure of technical staff, as well as the requirement to regularly clean equipment. Mannitol dry powder produced using spray drying to provide a uniform particle size, was found to be stable and suitable for encapsulation.[47] The pre-prepared package of mannitol provides a common operating standard for BPTs, with potential to compare results in different laboratories.

Following the establishment of reproducible baseline spirometry, the mannitol test requires the patient to inhale increasing doses of dry powder mannitol and have the FEV_1 measured in duplicate 60 seconds after each dose. The test protocol consists of 0-mg (empty capsule), 5-mg, 10-mg, 20-mg, 40-mg, and 80-mg (2×40-mg) capsules, and 3 doses of 160 mg (4×40-mg capsules) of mannitol. The maximum cumulative dose of mannitol that is administered is 635 mg.

A positive test result is defined as either a fall in FEV_1 of 15% from baseline (ie, post 0-mg capsule) or a 10% fall in FEV_1 from baseline between 2 consecutive doses.[34] If a patient presenting with symptoms suggestive of EIB has a fall of greater than 10% but less than 15% following the maximum cumulative dose of 635 mg (ie, only documenting a PD_{10}) then mild EIB could be considered[18] (see **Figs. 4** and **5**).

The mannitol test needs to be performed in a timely manner so that the osmotic gradient is increased with each dose. The repeatability of the PD_{15} to mannitol is 1 doubling-dose using a low-resistance dry powder inhaler.[47,48] The time to complete a positive test as observed in a large Phase 3 trial was 17 minutes (± 7 minutes) for a positive test, and 26 minutes (± 6 minutes) for a negative test.[23] A test taking more than 35 minutes may lead to a false-negative result.

SUMMARY AND FUTURE INVESTIGATIONS

Guidelines now recommend that EIB should be objectively identified using indirect BPTs, such as exercise, EVH, and mannitol, and not using direct tests, such as methacholine. Although laboratory exercise testing for EIB is appropriate and still useful, it has limitations when it comes to optimizing and standardizing both the exercise intensity and ambient conditions to produce a maximal dehydrating stimulus to the airways. EVH and osmotic stimuli, such as inhaling mannitol, have been used successfully in the laboratory for the diagnosis of asthma and EIB. The use of the surrogate tests has overcome many of the practical limitations in performing laboratory exercise, providing better standardization of procedures and improved diagnostic sensitivity.

REFERENCES

1. Weiler JM, Brannan JD, Randolph CC, et al. Exercise-induced bronchoconstriction update-2016. J Allergy Clin Immunol 2016;138(5):1292-5.
2. Weiler JM, Bonini S, Coifman R, et al. American Academy of Allergy, Asthma & Immunology Work Group report: exercise-induced asthma. J Allergy Clin Immunol 2007;119(6):1349-58.
3. Freed R, Anderson SD, Wyndham J. The use of bronchial provocation tests for identifying asthma. A review of the problems for occupational assessment and a proposal for a new direction. ADF Health 2002;3(2):77-85.
4. Miedinger D, Chhajed PN, Tamm M, et al. Diagnostic tests for asthma in firefighters. Chest 2007;131(6):1760-7.
5. Miedinger D, Blauenstein A, Wolf N, et al. Evaluation of fitness to utilize self-contained breathing apparatus (SCBA). J Asthma 2010;47(2):178-84.
6. Anderson SD, Lambert S, Brannan JD, et al. Laboratory protocol for exercise asthma to evaluate salbutamol given by two devices. Med Sci Sports Exerc 2001;33(6):893-900.
7. Godfrey S, Silverman M, Anderson SD. The use of the treadmill for assessing exercise-induced asthma and the effect of varying the severity and the duration of exercise. Paediatrics 1975;56(5(Pt 2)):893S-8S.
8. Haby MM, Anderson SD, Peat JK, et al. An exercise challenge protocol for epidemiological studies of asthma in children: comparison with histamine challenge. Eur Respir J 1994;7:43-9.
9. van Leeuwen JC, Driessen JM, de Jongh FH, et al. Measuring breakthrough exercise-induced bronchoconstriction in young asthmatic children using a jumping castle. J Allergy Clin Immunol 2013;131(5):1427-9.e5.
10. Argyros GJ, Roach JM, Hurwitz KM, et al. Eucapnic voluntary hyperventilation as a bronchoprovocation technique. Development of a standardized dosing schedule in asthmatics. Chest 1996;109:1520-4.
11. Anderson SD, Brannan JD. Methods for 'indirect' challenge tests including exercise, eucapnic voluntary hyperpnea and hypertonic aerosols. Clin Rev Allergy Immunol 2003;24:63-90.
12. Anderson SD. 'Indirect' challenges from science to clinical practice. Eur Clin Respir J 2016;3:31096.
13. O'Sullivan S, Roquet A, Dahlen B, et al. Evidence for mast cell activation during exercise-induced bronchoconstriction. Eur Respir J 1988;12(2):345-50.
14. Brannan JD, Gulliksson M, Anderson SD, et al. Evidence of mast cell activation and leukotriene release after mannitol inhalation. Eur Respir J 2003;22(3):491-6.
15. Kippelen P, Larsson J, Anderson SD, et al. Effect of sodium cromoglycate on mast cell mediators during hyperpnea in athletes. Med Sci Sports Exerc 2010;42(10):1853-60.
16. Mickleborough TD, Murray RL, Ionescu AA, et al. Fish oil supplementation reduces severity of exercise-induced bronchoconstriction in elite athletes. Am J Respir Crit Care Med 2003;168(10):1181-9.
17. Brannan JD, Koskela H, Anderson SD, et al. Responsiveness to mannitol in asthmatic subjects with exercise- and hyperventilation-induced asthma. Am J Respir Crit Care Med 1998;158(4):1120-6.
18. Holzer K, Anderson SD, Chan H-K, et al. Mannitol as a challenge test to identify exercise-induced bronchoconstriction in elite athletes. Am J Respir Crit Care Med 2003;167(4):534-47.

19. Elkins MR, Brannan JD. Warm-up exercise can reduce exercise-induced bronchoconstriction. Br J Sports Med 2013;47(10):657–8.
20. Coates AL, Wanger J, Cockcroft DW, et al. ERS technical standard on bronchial challenge testing: general considerations and performance of methacholine challenge tests. Eur Respir J 2017;49(5) [pii:1601526].
21. Cockcroft DW. Direct challenge tests: airway hyperresponsiveness in asthma: its measurement and clinical significance. Chest 2010;138(2 Suppl):18S–24S.
22. Backer V, Ulrik CS. Bronchial responsiveness to exercise in a random sample of 494 children and adolescents from Copenhagen. Clin Exp Allergy 1992;22: 741–7.
23. Anderson SD, Charlton B, Weiler JM, et al. Comparison of mannitol and methacholine to predict exercise-induced bronchoconstriction and a clinical diagnosis of asthma. Respir Res 2009;10:4.
24. Holley AB, Cohee B, Walter RJ, et al. Eucapnic voluntary hyperventilation is superior to methacholine challenge testing for detecting airway hyperreactivity in non-athletes. J Asthma 2012;49(6):614–9.
25. O'Byrne PM. Leukotrienes in the pathogenesis of asthma. Chest 1997;111(Suppl 2):27S–34S.
26. Anderson SD, Kippelen P. Assessment of EIB: what you need to know to optimize test results. Immunol Allergy Clin North Am 2013;33(3):363–80, viii.
27. Anderson SD. Single-dose agents in the prevention of exercise-induced asthma: a descriptive review. Treat Respir Med 2004;3(6):365–79.
28. Anderson SD, Pearlman DS, Rundell KW, et al. Reproducibility of the airway response to an exercise protocol standardized for intensity, duration, and inspired air conditions, in subjects with symptoms suggestive of asthma. Respir Res 2010;11:120.
29. Price OJ, Ansley L, Hull JH. Diagnosing exercise-induced bronchoconstriction with eucapnic voluntary hyperpnea: is one test enough? J Allergy Clin Immunol Pract 2015;3(2):243–9.
30. Mannix ET, Manfredi F, Farber MO. A comparison of two challenge tests for identifying exercise-induced bronchospasm in figure skaters. Chest 1999;115: 649–53.
31. Rundell KW, Anderson SD, Spiering BA, et al. Field exercise vs laboratory eucapnic voluntary hyperventilation to identify airway hyperresponsiveness in elite cold weather athletes. Chest 2004;125:909–15.
32. Dickinson J. Screening elite winter athletes for exercise induced asthma: a comparison of three challenge methods. Br J Sports Med 2006;40(2):179–82.
33. Purokivi M, Koskela H, Brannan JD, et al. Cough response to isocapnic hyperpnoea of dry air and hypertonic saline are interrelated. Cough 2011;7(1):8.
34. Brannan JD, Anderson SD, Perry CP, et al. The safety and efficacy of inhaled dry powder mannitol as a bronchial provocation test for airway hyperresponsiveness: a phase 3 comparison study with hypertonic (4.5%) saline. Respir Res 2005;6:144.
35. Koskela HO, Hyvärinen L, Brannan JD, et al. Coughing during mannitol challenge is associated with asthma. Chest 2004;125(6):1985–92.
36. Parsons JP, Hallstrand TS, Mastronarde JG, et al. An official American Thoracic Society clinical practice guideline: exercise-induced bronchoconstriction. Am J Respir Crit Care Med 2013;187(9):1016–27.
37. Dahlén B, O'Byrne PM, Watson RM, et al. The reproducibility and sample size requirements of exercise-induced bronchoconstriction measurements. Eur Respir J 2001;17(4):581–8.

38. Anderson SD, Daviskas E. The mechanism of exercise-induced asthma is .... J Allergy Clin Immunol 2000;106(3):453–9.
39. Phillips YY, Jaeger JJ, Laube BL, et al. Eucapnic voluntary hyperventilation of compressed gas mixture. A simple system for bronchial challenge by respiratory heat loss. Am Rev Respir Dis 1985;131:31–5.
40. O'Cain CF, Hensley MJ, McFadden ER Jr, et al. Pattern and mechanism of airway response to hypocapnia in normal subjects. J Appl Physiol Respir Environ Exerc Physiol 1979;47(1):8–12.
41. EucapSYS system for eucapnic voluntary hyperpnea, 2014. 2014. SMTEC sports and medical technologies Web site. Available at: http://www.smtech.net. Accessed May 1, 2017.
42. Smith CM, Anderson SD, Seale JP. The duration of action of the combination of fenoterol hydrobromide and ipratropium bromide in protecting against asthma provoked by hyperpnea. Chest 1988;94:709–17.
43. Price OJ, Ansley L, Levai IK, et al. Eucapnic voluntary hyperpnea testing in asymptomatic athletes. Am J Respir Crit Care Med 2016;193(10):1178–80.
44. Stadelmann K, Stensrud T, Carlsen KH. Respiratory symptoms and bronchial responsiveness in competitive swimmers. Med Sci Sports Exerc 2011;43(3): 375–81.
45. Williams NC, Johnson MA, Hunter KA, et al. Reproducibility of the bronchoconstrictive response to eucapnic voluntary hyperpnoea. Respir Med 2015; 109(10):1262–7.
46. Aridol; mannitol bronchial challenge test, 2017. 2017. Pharmaxis Ltd Web site for aridol. Available at: http://www.aridol.info. Accessed May 1, 2017.
47. Anderson SD, Brannan J, Spring J, et al. A new method for bronchial-provocation testing in asthmatic subjects using a dry powder of mannitol. Am J Respir Crit Care Med 1997;156:758–65.
48. Brannan JD, Anderson SD, Gomes K, et al. Fexofenadine decreases sensitivity to and montelukast improves recovery from inhaled mannitol. Am J Respir Crit Care Med 2001;163:1420–5.

Pharmacologic Strategies for Exercise-Induced Bronchospasm with a Focus on Athletes

Vibeke Backer, MD, DMSci[a],*, John Mastronarde, MD, MSc[b]

KEYWORDS

- Exercise • Asthma • Treatment • EIB • Doping

KEY POINTS

- Short-acting beta agonists are effective first-line agents for exercise-induced broncho-spasm (EIB). Tolerance can develop with frequent use.
- Multiple other medication classes are effective in the treatment of EIB, and selection of these agents can be stratified by the presence or absence of underlying asthma and the frequency of short-acting beta-agonist use.
- In the future, therapy may be guided by the identification of one or more specific EIB endo-types.
- Lack of specific data regarding EIB in elite athletes results in recommendations for treatment strategies that are similar to EIB in nonathletes.
- Athletes and providers must be cognizant of the World Anti-Doping Agency's regulations with regard to EIB therapy in elite athletes.

INTRODUCTION

Exercise-induced bronchoconstriction (EIB) is the transient narrowing of the airways during and after exercise that occurs in response to increased ventilation in susceptible individuals.[1] EIB is a common phenomenon affecting as many as 20% of the general population and most of the estimated 300 million patients with asthma worldwide.[2,3] Among athletes, as reviewed by Matteo Bonini and William Silvers (See Matteo Bonini

Disclosure Statement: None of the authors has anything to disclose or any conflicts of interest. V. Backer has received support from the World Anti-Doping Agency for asthma therapy evaluation in elite athletes.

[a] Department of Respiratory Medicine, Bispebjerg Hospital, University of Copenhagen, Bispebjerg Bakke 23, Copenhagen NV 2400, Denmark; [b] Department of Medical Education, Providence Portland Medical Center, Pulmonary/Critical Care Medicine, Oregon Health & Science University, 5050 Northeast Hoyt Avenue, Suite 540, Portland, OR 97213, USA
* Corresponding author.
E-mail address: backer@dadlnet.dk

and William Silvers's article, "Exercise-Induced Bronchoconstriction: Background, Prevalence, and Sport Considerations," in this issue.) and others, the prevalence can be much higher depending on specific sport requirements; dry ambient conditions are known to contribute.[4–8] The impact of the condition manifests in several very important ways, including the potential for EIB to do the following:

1. To theoretically cause changes in airway function[9–11]
2. To act as a deterrent to exercise in an age when exercise is promoted as a therapy for many health conditions[12–15]
3. To negatively affect sport performance in competitive athletes[16]

For all of these reasons, bronchospasm that occurs in isolation with exercise or as a manifestation of chronic asthma is important to treat.

This review of EIB therapeutics relates pharmacologic interventions to known elements of disease mechanism and includes a discussion of EIB in patients with and without underlying asthma (EIBa and EIBwa, respectively) with an assumption that other causes of exertional cough and dyspnea, including exercise-induced laryngeal obstruction, have been excluded. As with most diseases, our knowledge of the mechanism exceeds the availability of pharmacologic agents that can effectively target important molecular or cellular intermediaries of the disease. Pascale Kippelen and colleagues (See Pascale Kippelen and colleagues' article, "Mechanisms and Biomarkers of Exercise-Induced Bronchoconstriction," in this issue.) thoroughly review the current knowledge regarding the disease mechanism, calling attention to the isolation of EIBwa as a distinct endo-type of asthma.[17–19] Extending this line of thinking, it is possible that multiple endo-types of EIBwa exist with varying inflammatory profiles and may be supported by decades of observations of differential responses to medication across subjects.[20,21] Kenneth W. Rundell and colleagues (see Kenneth W. Rundell and colleagues' article, "Exercise-Induced Bronchoconstriction and the Air We Breathe," in this issue.) thoroughly review environmental factors that could also modulate the molecular and cellular responses to increased ventilation during exercise acutely and chronically.[22]

In this review, the authors summarize all of the medication classes that are commonly used in the treatment of EIB. The authors highlight specific benefits, drawbacks, and situational considerations of the medications as supported in the medical literature. In this process, the authors refer to consensus recommendations that have been recently published by the American Thoracic Society and the Joint Task Force on Practice Parameters representing the American Academy of Allergy, Asthma & Immunology, the American College of Allergy, Asthma & Immunology, and the Joint Council of Allergy, Asthma & Immunology.[23,24] The authors highlight important considerations with regard to the World Anti-Doping Agency's (WADA) current regulations.[25]

OVERVIEW OF PHARMACOLOGIC THERAPY FOR EXERCISE-INDUCED BRONCHOCONSTRICTION

Although molecular and clinical asthma literature increasingly discusses the use of asthma endo-types to guide therapy, at the current time, there is not literature that strongly recommends stratification of therapy across groups with potentially distinct inflammatory signatures with isolated EIBwa or across the larger groups of EIBa and EIBwa. For this reason, many of the observations and recommendations that follow can be considered for all patients who experience EIB. This approach is in line with recommendations from the recently published practice parameter and the International Olympic Committee's consensus conference on asthma and the elite athlete.[24,26] However, a personalized approach can guide EIB therapy for reasons unrelated to inflammatory signatures. As per current guidelines, such an approach should include concurrent evaluation and treatment of conditions extrinsic to isolated EIB that affect EIB, including nonallergic sino-nasal disease (See Brecht Steelant and colleagues' article, "Exercise and Sino-Nasal Disease," in this issue.), allergic disease, underlying asthma, exercise frequency, medication nonadherence, and poor medication delivery (the details of which are beyond the scope of this review).[27,28] This approach may also extend to considerations relevant to specific sports, including cold-weather endurance sports and swimming, that present unique challenges and daily training regimens, which could potentially induce bronchodilator tolerance.[29]

Beyond personalized recommendations, the authors discuss incremental therapy for patients who continue to experience symptoms despite appropriate monotherapy followed by a framework for approaching patients with difficult-to-manage symptoms. Although there are little experimental data to support individual steps in an incremental approach to EIB therapy, the stepwise approach outlined in the "Expert Panel Report 3"[27] for asthma management provides a useful therapy model.

Short-Acting Beta$_2$ Agonists: First-Line Therapy for Exercise-Induced Bronchoconstriction

Short-acting beta agonists (SABAs) should be considered the first-line agents for broncho-protection against EIB and acute bronchodilation in the treatment of EIB based on consistent results across multiple meta-analyses of head-to-head trials against all other classes of medications commonly used in the condition and consensus guidelines.[23,24,27,28,30,31] Typically, SABAs are administered 15 to 20 minutes before exercise in a dose of albuterol (salbutamol) 0.2 to 0.4 mg inhaled or terbutaline 0.5 to 1.0 mg inhaled. They have a rapid onset and duration of action of 2 to 4 hours.[32]

Although effective in most patients, multiple studies in both children and adults, using a variety of exercise challenges, indicate SABAs may not protect against EIB in roughly 15% to 20% of patients.[32–34] Chronic SABA administration may lead to tolerance, defined as a lack of broncho-protection or shortened duration of broncho-protection that occurs after repeated medication use, a phenomenon that affects treatment guidelines.[23,31] Hancox and colleagues,[35] in 2002, demonstrated that daily use of salbutamol for 6 to 10 days resulted in decreased broncho-protection to exercise challenge and delayed the response to salbutamol given after exercise as a rescue in 8 participants. Inman and O'Byrne[36] demonstrated a similar decrease in broncho-protection in 10 participants after 7 days of regular use of albuterol, although albuterol was effective after exercise in their trial. The mechanism for development of tolerance is suspected to be downregulation of beta$_{-2}$ receptors on mast cells and airway smooth muscle.[37] The clinical significance of SABA tolerance in athletes is unknown. Furthermore, the prevalence of tolerance among elite athletes and threshold dosing to induce tolerance are also unknown. Thus, the current guidelines suggest if SABAs are needed daily for EIB, an additional agent should be added to decrease the frequency of SABA use.[23] With respect to treatment of elite athletes, it is important to know that regulations change over time. The WADA's current regulations require therapeutic use exemptions (TUEs) for all selective and nonselective SABAs except inhaled albuterol (salbutamol, with a maximum dosage of 1600 µg over 24 hours or 800 µg over 12 hours).[25]

Alternative First-Line Therapies and Additions to Short-Acting Beta-Agonist Therapy

Inhaled corticosteroids

Inhaled corticosteroid (ICS) can be used as specific therapy for EIBa and EIBwa, with effectiveness associated with the duration of therapy and dosage. Although a single dose of ICS improves EIB airflow physiology,[38,39] the measured benefit of low-dose ICS increases incrementally to a plateau that may occur weeks after initiating therapy.[40,41] Increased broncho-protection has been measured with high-dose ciclesonide regimens when compared with low-dose regimens in a trial evaluating incremental doses.[41] With regard to the treatment of elite athletes, current (WADA) regulations permit the use of ICSs and require TUEs for oral, intravenous, intramuscular, and rectal administration of glucocorticoids.[25]

Long-acting beta₂ agonists

As SABAs did not resolve all symptoms in all patients, there is a need to understand alternative therapies for patients who are nonresponders to SABAs and adjunctive therapies for patients who are partially responsive. Long-acting beta₂ agonists (LABAs) have also been demonstrated to be protective for EIB with an expected longer duration of protection than SABAs,[32] but they are not to be used without an undelining inflammatory controller with inhaled steroid.[42–44] This tolerance is not diminished by adding ICS (**Fig. 1**).[45] As with chronic SABA use, the prevalence and impact of SABA tolerance in elite athletes using chronic LABAs are unknown. Concerns regarding serious adverse events associated with LABA use, specifically the increased risk of severe exacerbations and death, have led to recommendations that LABAs never be used as monotherapy for underlying asthma.[27,28] Given the nature of these potential events, the recommendation against LABA monotherapy is reflected in guidelines in the management of EIB.[23,24] With respect to the treatment of elite athletes, current (WADA) regulations require TUEs for all selective and nonselective LABAs except inhaled fomoterol (with a maximum dosage of 54 µg over 24 hours) and inhaled salmeterol (with a maximum dosage of 200 µg over 24 hours).[25]

Leukotriene receptor antagonists and 5-lipoxyenase inhibitors

As the cysteinyl leukotriene pathway has been demonstrated to be involved in the pathophysiology of EIB,[46,47] LTRAs have been studied for decades as monotherapy and adjunct therapy for EIB.

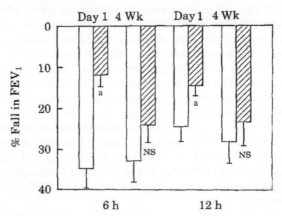

Fig. 1. Percentage decrease in forced expiratory volume in 1 second (FEV₁) after exercise challenge. NS, non significant. [a] Significant difference ($P<.05$) between salmeterol (▨), placebo (☐). (*From* Ramage L, Lipworth BJ, Ingram CG, et al. Reduced protection against exercise induced bronchoconstriction after chronic dosing with salmeterol. Respir Med 1994;88(5):363–8; with permission.)

Several trials have demonstrated efficacy after a single dose of montelukast given 1 to 2 hours before exercise with protection documented at 12 and 24 hours after dosing.[48,49] In a trial (of 10 subjects) evaluating multiple medications in these classes, single doses of montelukast, zafirlukast, and the 5-lipoxygenase inhibitor zileuton were all effective in preventing EIB.[50] Montelukast has been demonstrated to be effective in preventing EIB when used chronically without the development of tolerance, which is observed in patients chronically using SABAs and LABAs.[51,52] There are few studies of LTRAs in isolated populations of athletes. Montelukast protected against EIB in collegiate hockey players in low- and high-particulate-matter environments (**Fig. 2**).[53,54] With respect to the treatment of elite athletes, LTRAs and zileuton are both currently permitted under the WADA's regulations.[25]

MAST CELL STABILIZING AGENTS

Mast cell stabilizing agents (MCSAs), such as cromolyn or nedocromil, have been used for decades in the treatment of EIB because the mast cell is known to play an important role in the pathophysiology of EIB.[55] The investigators of a Cochrane review concluded that MCSAs are effective in the treatment of EIB when compared with placebo but less effective than SABAs when trialed head-to-head and ineffective when used as a therapy in addition to SABAs.[30] Although it is theoretically possible that specific subgroups of patients preferentially respond to MCSAs, the use of these agents is somewhat limited, as these medications are not available in all countries. With respect to the treatment of elite athletes, MCSAs are currently permitted under the WADA's regulations.[25]

ANTICHOLINERGIC AGENTS

Short-acting muscarinic antagonists (SAMAs), including ipratropium, which target muscarinic receptors on bronchial smooth muscle leading to relaxation and bronchodilation, are effective single agents when used for broncho-protection or bronchodilation in patients with EIB.[21,56,57] Ipratropium is not as effective as SABAs in terms of

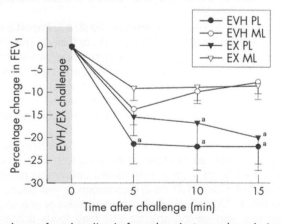

Fig. 2. Percentage change from baseline in forced expiratory volume in 1 second (FEV_1) 5, 10, and 15 minutes after the completion of eucapnic voluntary hyperventilation (EVH) and high-intensity 6-minute cycle ergometer challenge in cold-temperature-conditions (EX) trials on placebo (PL) and montelukast (ML) treatments. [a] Significant differences between placebo and montelukast for respective challenges at each time point. (*From* Rundell K, Spiering B, Baumann J, et al. Effects of montelukast on airway narrowing from eucapnic voluntary hyperventilation and cold air exercise. Br J Sports Med 2005;39(4):234; with permission.)

broncho-protective or bronchodilator activity; but it fills a clinical niche, as it maintains its effectiveness in patients with SABA tolerance given its alternative mechanism of action.[57,58] There are also data demonstrating an additive benefit of ipratropium to albuterol in terms of acute asthma symptom control outside of exercise.[59] There are not data evaluating the efficacy of long-acting muscarinic antagonists (LAMAs), including tiotropium, for broncho-protection in EIB, although the medication has been evaluated (with and without LABA) with respect to its effect on exercise tolerance in patients with chronic obstructive pulmonary disease.[60,61] With respect to treatment of elite athletes, SAMAs and LAMAs are currently permitted under the WADA's regulations.[25]

SCIENTIFIC EXPERIENCE WITH MULTIDRUG THERAPY FOR EXERCISE-INDUCED BRONCHOCONSTRICTION

Clinical experience and experimental evidence suggests that there is a need to develop treatment strategies for patients who continue to struggle with symptoms of EIB despite the use of albuterol as a broncho-protective agent in EIBa and EIBwa.[32] However, definitive evidence favoring specific agents for add-on therapy to SABA is scant because there are notable challenges to implementation of clinical trials designed to identify the relative effectiveness of SABA therapy adjuncts in EIB, including variability in measured bronchoconstriction across time within subjects, stratification of subjects based on the presence of EIBa versus EIBwa, and the effectiveness of SABAs. Given the lack of direct evidence, practice patterns may be driven by indirect evidence, including the effectiveness of controller therapy regimens in patients with baseline asthma against bronchoconstriction caused as a result of exercise or surrogate challenge (performed without SABA broncho-protection).[62–64]

APPROACH TO PATIENTS WITH DIFFICULT-TO-MANAGE EXERCISE-INDUCED BRONCHOCONSTRICTION

As experimental evidence is lacking regarding selection of the best add-on therapy to SABAs for the treatment of confirmed EIB, clinicians must interpret and prioritize related information.

The authors recommend 2 initial assessments. First, it is important to characterize patients who require add-on therapy as having EIBa or EIBwa. This decision is important because current guidelines suggest that clinicians view persistent exercise symptoms in patients with EIBa as a reflection of poorly controlled underlying asthma.[27] Secondly, it is important to characterize exercise frequency as daily versus less frequent. The reasoning behind this stratification is related to the development of SABA tolerance and guideline recommendations to institute add-on therapy in patients requiring daily SABAs.[23]

In patients with EIBwa, it is especially important to determine exercise frequency and SABA use frequency with an eye toward avoiding tolerance. In patients who exercise daily and use SABAs daily (or more), recent consensus panels have strongly supported the addition of ICSs.[23] LTRAs are an option as well based on these guidelines in this circumstance.[23] In patients who do not exercise or use SABAs daily, recent guidelines suggest that add-on therapy for EIB may focus primarily on broncho-protection before exercise. In this case, the addition of SAMAs or MCSAs is a reasonable option.[23]

In patients with EIBa and frequent EIB symptoms, the current guidelines strongly recommend the initiation of inhaled steroids as an initial daily therapy.[27,28] With respect to underlying asthma, ICSs reduce mortality, exacerbation frequency, exacerbation severity, symptoms, and airway inflammation and improve lung function and quality of life.[65–68] Although a detailed review of baseline asthma management is beyond the scope of this review, step-up therapy options from low-dose ICSs include the addition of LABAs, LTRAs, or transition to medium-dose ICSs.[27,69] Tiotropium has also been studied in adults as an add-on therapy in moderate asthma management.[70,71] When clinicians are treating patients with EIBa who perform daily exercise in whom step-up from low-dose ICSs is indicated, it is rational to consider moderate-dose ICSs preferentially over ICS/LABA combinations in order to avoid SABA tolerance.[41] This theoretic benefit must be weighed against the documented decrements in linear growth velocity and adult height that accompany incremental increases in inhaled steroid usage in children and adolescents.[72] It is important to note that there is not experimental evidence that confirms the effectiveness of this approach. A decision tree graphically representing this logic is reproduced (**Fig. 3**).

EXERCISE-INDUCED BRONCHOCONSTRICTION THERAPY STRATIFIED BY ENDO-TYPE

As our ability to characterize the biology of patients improves, it is possible to envision EIB therapy decision trees based on inflammatory profiles or other biological parameters that can be linked to a distinct mechanism. A pilot trial for this type of decision-making has been completed in patients with mild intermittent asthma (which is not synonymous with EIBwa).[20] In this trial, subjects demonstrated a differential EIB response to incremental doses of ICS, with the response associated with steroid-

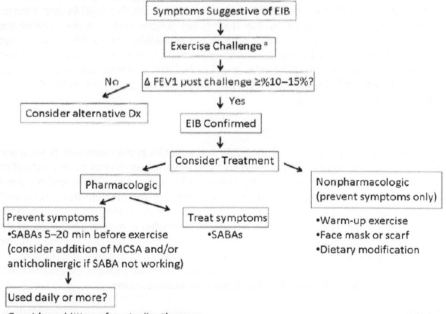

Fig. 3. Diagnostic and treatment algorithm for EIB. Dx, diagnosis. [a] Or surrogate challenge, for example, hyperpnea or mannitol. (*From* Parsons JP, Hallstrand TS, Mastronarde JG, et al. An Official American Thoracic Society Clinical Practice Guideline: Exercise-induced Bronchoconstriction. Am J Respir Crit Care Med 2013;187(9):1018; Reprinted with permission of the American Thoracic Society. Copyright © 2018 American Thoracic Society. The American Journal of Respiratory and Critical Care Medicine is an official journal of the American Thoracic Society.)

naïve sputum eosinophil counts. Subjects with sputum eosinophil counts greater than 5% responded to the low-dose ICS (defined as an experiencing a decrease in postexercise decrement in forced expiratory volume in 1 second [FEV_1]), with an enhanced response to a high-dose ICS. Subjects with sputum eosinophil counts less than 5% also responded to a low-dose ICS but did not show an enhanced response to a high-dose ICS.

Elite Nordic skiers may have a different inflammatory phenotype than other patients with EIBa or EIBwa, with a notably low eosinophil count.[18,73] Currently, there are no specific data that favor a specific medication strategy in this group of patients. Future clinical trials of SAMAs and LAMAs may be warranted in Nordic skiers with EIB based on the experimental observation that elite athletes in general have increased vagal tone compared with population controls.[74]

TREATMENT OF ACUTE EXACERBATION IN ELITE ATHLETES AND THE DOPING PERSPECTIVE

Athletes with asthma and the providers who are responsible for medication prescription must be cognizant of the WADA's regulations that are relevant to asthma exacerbations, defined by symptomatic or physiologic criteria.[75] As with all patients, there are strong recommendations to treat asthma exacerbations with oral steroids and increases in bronchodilators.[27] However, it is important to note that the use of oral, intramuscular, intravenous, and rectal corticosteroids requires a TUE under the WADA's current regulations.[25] With respect to bronchodilators, inhaled SABAs and inhaled LABAs are permitted, subject to the dosing restrictions noted earlier, under the WADA's current regulations.[25] Urinary measures of SABAs and LABAs that exceed threshold levels thought to correlate with maximal inhaled dosing are considered adverse analytical findings.[25] SAMAs and LAMAs are currently permitted per the WADA's regulations.[25] Further specific information is available online at the following address: www.globaldro.org.

SUMMARY

Several pharmacologic agents are available and effective in the treatment of EIBa and EIBwa, with SABAs demonstrating head-to-head advantages over all other medication classes. An estimated 15% of patients suboptimally respond to SABAs and require a second agent to manage the disease. In these situations, and the authors recommend, stratifying treatment based on the presence or absence of underlying asthma and the frequency of exercise and SABA use, a strategy promoted in recent guidelines. In the future, stratification may be driven by endo-typic characterization of patients. Athletes with EIB and their health care providers must be cognizant of the WADA's regulations, which can change over time and currently mandate TUEs for multiple classes of medications used in the treatment of EIB and asthma exacerbations.

REFERENCES

1. Jones RS, Buston MH, Wharton MJ. The effect of exercise on ventilatory function in the child with asthma. Br J Dis Chest 1962;56:78–86.
2. Mannix ET, Roberts M, Fagin DP, et al. The prevalence of airways hyperresponsiveness in members of an exercise training facility. J Asthma 2003;40(4):349–55.
3. Masoli M, Fabian D, Holt S, et al, Global Initiative for Asthma (GINA) Program. The global burden of asthma: executive summary of the GINA Dissemination Committee report. Allergy 2004;59(5):469–78.

4. Carlsen KH, Anderson SD, Bjermer L, et al. Exercise-induced asthma, respiratory and allergic disorders in elite athletes: epidemiology, mechanisms and diagnosis: part I of the report from the Joint Task Force of the European Respiratory Society (ERS) and the European Academy of Allergy and Clinical Immunology (EAACI) in cooperation with GA2LEN. Allergy 2008;63(4):387–403.

5. Wilber RL, Rundell KW, Szmedra L, et al. Incidence of exercise-induced bronchospasm in Olympic winter sport athletes. Med Sci Sports Exerc 2000;32(4):732–7.

6. Stensrud T, Berntsen S, Carlsen KH. Humidity influences exercise capacity in subjects with exercise-induced bronchoconstriction (EIB). Respir Med 2006; 100(9):1633–41.

7. Stensrud T, Berntsen S, Carlsen KH. Exercise capacity and exercise-induced bronchoconstriction (EIB) in a cold environment. Respir Med 2007;101(7): 1529–36.

8. Burns J, Mason C, Mueller N, et al. Asthma prevalence in Olympic summer athletes and the general population: an analysis of three European countries. Respir Med 2015;109(7):813–20.

9. Helenius I, Rytila P, Sarna S, et al. Effect of continuing or finishing high-level sports on airway inflammation, bronchial hyperresponsiveness, and asthma: a 5-year prospective follow-up study of 42 highly trained swimmers. J Allergy Clin Immunol 2002;109(6):962–8.

10. Eslami-Behroozi M, Pazhoohan S, Aref E, et al. Bronchoconstriction induces structural and functional airway alterations in non-sensitized rats. Lung 2017; 195(2):167–71.

11. Grainge CL, Lau LC, Ward JA, et al. Effect of bronchoconstriction on airway remodeling in asthma. N Engl J Med 2011;364(21):2006–15.

12. World Health Organization. Global recommendations on physical activity for health. 2017. Available at: http://apps.who.int/iris/bitstream/10665/44399/1/9789241599979_eng.pdf.

13. Vahlkvist S, Pedersen S. Fitness, daily activity and body composition in children with newly diagnosed, untreated asthma. Allergy 2009;64(11):1649–55.

14. Glazebrook C, McPherson AC, Macdonald IA, et al. Asthma as a barrier to children's physical activity: implications for body mass index and mental health. Pediatrics 2006;118(6):2443–9.

15. Dantas FM, Correia MA Jr, Silva AR, et al. Mothers impose physical activity restrictions on their asthmatic children and adolescents: an analytical cross-sectional study. BMC Public Health 2014;14(1):287.

16. Price OJ, Hull JH, Backer V, et al. The impact of exercise-induced bronchoconstriction on athletic performance: a systematic review. Sports Med 2014;44(12): 1749–61.

17. Lai Y, Altemeier WA, Vandree J, et al. Increased density of intraepithelial mast cells in patients with exercise-induced bronchoconstriction regulated through epithelially derived thymic stromal lymphopoietin and IL-33. J Allergy Clin Immunol 2014;133(5):1448–55.

18. Lotvall J, Akdis CA, Bacharier LB, et al. Asthma endotypes: a new approach to classification of disease entities within the asthma syndrome. J Allergy Clin Immunol 2011;127(2):355–60.

19. Wenzel SE. Asthma phenotypes: the evolution from clinical to molecular approaches. Nat Med 2012;18(5):716–25.

20. Duong M, Subbarao P, Adelroth E, et al. Sputum eosinophils and the response of exercise-induced bronchoconstriction to corticosteroid in asthma. Chest 2008; 133(2):404–11.

21. Chan-Yeung M. The effect of Sch 1000 and disodium cromoglycate on exercise-induced asthma. Chest 1977;71(3):320–3.

22. Salvi S, Blomberg A, Rudell B, et al. Acute inflammatory responses in the airways and peripheral blood after short-term exposure to diesel exhaust in healthy human volunteers. Am J Respir Crit Care Med 1999;159(3):702–9.

23. Parsons JP, Hallstrand TS, Mastronarde JG, et al. An official American Thoracic Society clinical practice guideline: exercise-induced bronchoconstriction. Am J Respir Crit Care Med 2013;187(9):1016–27.

24. Weiler JM, Brannan JD, Randolph CC, et al. Exercise-induced bronchoconstriction update-2016. J Allergy Clin Immunol 2016;138(5):1292–5.e36.

25. World Anti-Doping Agency. The world anti-doping code international standard. Prohibited list: January, 2017. 2017. Available at: https://www.wada-ama.org/sites/default/files/resources/files/2016-09-29_-_wada_prohibited_list_2017_eng_final.pdf. Accessed June 27, 2017.

26. Fitch KD, Sue-Chu M, Anderson SD, et al. Asthma and the elite athlete: summary of the International Olympic Committee's consensus conference, Lausanne, Switzerland, January 22-24, 2008. J Allergy Clin Immunol 2008;122(2):254–60, 260.e1-7.

27. National Asthma Education and Prevention Program. Expert panel report 3 (EPR-3): guidelines for the diagnosis and management of asthma-summary report 2007. J Allergy Clin Immunol 2007;120(5 Suppl):S94–138.

28. Reddel HK, Bateman ED, Becker A, et al. A summary of the new GINA strategy: a roadmap to asthma control. Eur Respir J 2015;46(3):622–39.

29. Sue-Chu M, Larsson L, Moen T, et al. Bronchoscopy and bronchoalveolar lavage findings in cross-country skiers with and without "ski asthma". Eur Respir J 1999; 13(3):626–32.

30. Spooner C, Spooner GR, Rowe BH. Mast-cell stabilising agents to prevent exercise-induced bronchoconstriction. Cochrane Database Syst Rev 2003;(4):CD002307.

31. Carlsen KH, Anderson SD, Bjermer L, et al. Treatment of exercise-induced asthma, respiratory and allergic disorders in sports and the relationship to doping: part II of the report from the Joint Task Force of European Respiratory Society (ERS) and European Academy of Allergy and Clinical Immunology (EAACI) in cooperation with GA(2)LEN. Allergy 2008;63(5):492–505.

32. Anderson SD, Rodwell L, Du Toit J, et al. Duration of protection by inhaled salmeterol in exercise-induced asthma. Chest 1991;100(5):1254–60.

33. Anderson SD, Caillaud C, Brannan JD. β2-agonists and exercise-induced asthma. Clin Rev Allergy Immunol 2006;31(2–3):163–80.

34. Bonini M, Di Mambro C, Calderon MA, et al. Beta2-agonists for exercise-induced asthma. Cochrane Database Syst Rev 2013;(10):CD003564.

35. Hancox RJ, Subbarao P, Kamada D, et al. β2-agonist tolerance and exercise-induced bronchospasm. Am J Respir Crit Care Med 2002;165(8):1068–70.

36. Inman MD, O'Byrne PM. The effect of regular inhaled albuterol on exercise-induced bronchoconstriction. Am J Respir Crit Care Med 1996;153(1):65–9.

37. Finney PA, Belvisi MG, Donnelly LE, et al. Albuterol-induced downregulation of Gsα accounts for pulmonary β(2)-adrenoceptor desensitization in vivo. J Clin Invest 2000;106(1):125–35.

38. Kippelen P, Larsson J, Anderson SD, et al. Acute effects of beclomethasone on hyperpnea-induced bronchoconstriction. Med Sci Sports Exerc 2010;42(2):273–80.

39. Driessen J, Nieland H, van der Palen JAM, et al. Effects of a single dose inhaled corticosteroid on the dynamics of airway obstruction after exercise. Pediatr Pulmonol 2011;46(9):849–56.

40. Hofstra WB, Neijens HJ, Duiverman EJ, et al. Dose-responses over time to inhaled fluticasone propionate treatment of exercise- and methacholine-induced bronchoconstriction in children with asthma. Pediatr Pulmonol 2000; 29(6):415–23.

41. Subbarao P, Duong M, Adelroth E, et al. Effect of ciclesonide dose and duration of therapy on exercise-induced bronchoconstriction in patients with asthma. J Allergy Clin Immunol 2006;117(5):1008–13.

42. Villaran C, O'Neill SJ, Helbling A, et al. Montelukast versus salmeterol in patients with asthma and exercise-induced bronchoconstriction. J Allergy Clin Immunol 1999;104(3):547–53.

43. Elers J, Strandbygaard U, Pedersen L, et al. Daily use of salmeterol causes tolerance to bronchodilation with terbutaline in asthmatic subjects. Open Respir Med J 2010;4:48.

44. Ramage L, Lipworth B, Ingram C, et al. Reduced protection against exercise induced bronchoconstriction after chronic dosing with salmeterol. Respir Med 1994;88(5):363–8.

45. Simons FER, Gerstner TV, Cheang MS. Tolerance to the bronchoprotective effect of salmeterol in adolescents with exercise-induced asthma using concurrent inhaled glucocorticoid treatment. Pediatrics 1997;99(5):655–9.

46. Kikawa Y, Miyanomae T, Inoue Y, et al. Urinary leukotriene E 4 after exercise challenge in children with asthma. J Allergy Clin Immunol 1992;89(6):1111–9.

47. Reiss TF, Hill JB, Harman E, et al. Increased urinary excretion of LTE4 after exercise and attenuation of exercise-induced bronchospasm by montelukast, a cysteinyl leukotriene receptor antagonist. Thorax 1997;52(12):1030–5.

48. Pearlman DS, van Adelsberg J, Philip G, et al. Onset and duration of protection against exercise-induced bronchoconstriction by a single oral dose of montelukast. Ann Allergy Asthma Immunol 2006;97(1):98–104.

49. Philip G, Pearlman DS, Villarán C, et al. Single-dose montelukast or salmeterol as protection against exercise-induced bronchoconstriction. Chest 2007;132(3): 875–83.

50. Coreno A, Skowronski M, Kotaru C, et al. Comparative effects of long-acting β 2-agonists, leukotriene receptor antagonists, and a 5-lipoxygenase inhibitor on exercise-induced asthma. J Allergy Clin Immunol 2000;106(3):500–6.

51. de Benedictis FM, del Giudice MM, Forenza N, et al. Lack of tolerance to the protective effect of montelukast in exercise-induced bronchoconstriction in children. Eur Respir J 2006;28(2):291–5.

52. Leff JA, Busse WW, Pearlman D, et al. Montelukast, a leukotriene-receptor antagonist, for the treatment of mild asthma and exercise-induced bronchoconstriction. N Engl J Med 1998;339(3):147–52.

53. Rundell K, Spiering B, Baumann J, et al. Effects of montelukast on airway narrowing from eucapnic voluntary hyperventilation and cold air exercise. Br J Sports Med 2005;39(4):232–6.

54. Rundell KW, Spiering BA, Baumann JM, et al. Bronchoconstriction provoked by exercise in a high-particulate-matter environment is attenuated by montelukast. Inhal Toxicol 2005;17(2):99–105.

55. O'Sullivan S, Roquet A, Dahlen B, et al. Evidence for mast cell activation during exercise-induced bronchoconstriction. Eur Respir J 1998;12(2):345–50.

56. Thomson N, Patel K, Kerr J. Sodium cromoglycate and ipratropium bromide in exercise-induced asthma. Thorax 1978;33(6):694–9.

57. Boulet L-P, Turcotte H, Tennina S. Comparative efficacy of salbutamol, ipratropium, and cromoglycate in the prevention of bronchospasm induced by exercise and hyperosmolar challenges. J Allergy Clin Immunol 1989;83(5):882–7.

58. Haney S, Hancox RJ. Overcoming beta-agonist tolerance: high dose salbutamol and ipratropium bromide. Two randomised controlled trials. Respir Res 2007; 8(1):19.

59. Donohue JF, Wise R, Busse WW, et al. Efficacy and safety of ipratropium bromide/albuterol compared with albuterol in patients with moderate-to-severe asthma: a randomized controlled trial. BMC Pulm Med 2016;16(1):65.

60. O'Donnell DE, Casaburi R, Frith P, et al. Effects of combined tiotropium/olodaterol on inspiratory capacity and exercise endurance in COPD. Eur Respir J 2017; 49(4) [pii:1601348].

61. O'Donnell DE, Flüge T, Gerken F, et al. Effects of tiotropium on lung hyperinflation, dyspnoea and exercise tolerance in COPD. Eur Respir J 2004;23(6):832–40.

62. Stelmach I, Grzelewski T, Majak P, et al. Effect of different antiasthmatic treatments on exercise-induced bronchoconstriction in children with asthma. J Allergy Clin Immunol 2008;121(2):383–9.

63. Duong M, Amin R, Baatjes AJ, et al. The effect of montelukast, budesonide alone, and in combination on exercise-induced bronchoconstriction. J Allergy Clin Immunol 2012;130(2):535–9.e3.

64. Weiler JM, Nathan RA, Rupp NT, et al. Effect of fluticasone/salmeterol administered via a single device on exercise-induced bronchospasm in patients with persistent asthma. Ann Allergy Asthma Immunol 2005;94(1):65–72.

65. Suissa S, Ernst P, Benayoun S, et al. Low-dose inhaled corticosteroids and the prevention of death from asthma. N Engl J Med 2000;343:332–6.

66. Jeffery P, Godfrey R, Ädelroth E, et al. Effects of treatment on airway inflammation and thickening of basement membrane reticular collagen in asthma: a quantitative light and electron microscopic study. Am Rev Respir Dis 1992;145(4_pt_1): 890–9.

67. O'Byrne PM, Barnes PJ, Rodriguez-Roisin R, et al. Low dose inhaled budesonide and formoterol in mild persistent asthma: the OPTIMA randomized trial. Am J Respir Crit Care Med 2001;164(8):1392–7.

68. Haahtela T, Järvinen M, Kava T, et al. Comparison of a β2-agonist, terbutaline, with an inhaled corticosteroid, budesonide, in newly detected asthma. N Engl J Med 1991;325(6):388–92.

69. Lemanske RF Jr, Mauger DT, Sorkness CA, et al. Step-up therapy for children with uncontrolled asthma receiving inhaled corticosteroids. N Engl J Med 2010; 362(11):975–85.

70. Kerstjens HAM, Casale TB, Bleecker ER, et al. Tiotropium or salmeterol as add-on therapy to inhaled corticosteroids for patients with moderate symptomatic asthma: two replicate, double-blind, placebo-controlled, parallel-group, active-comparator, randomised trials. Lancet Respir Med 2015;3(5):367–76.

71. Evans DJW, Kew KM, Anderson DE, et al. Long-acting muscarinic antagonists (LAMA) added to inhaled corticosteroids (ICS) versus higher dose ICS for adults with asthma. Cochrane Database Syst Rev 2015;(7):CD011437.

72. Kelly HW, Sternberg AL, Lescher R, et al. Effect of inhaled glucocorticoids in childhood on adult height. N Engl J Med 2012;367(10):904–12.

73. Sue-Chu M, Karjalainen EM, Laitinen A, et al. Placebo-controlled study of inhaled budesonide on indices of airway inflammation in bronchoalveolar lavage fluid and bronchial biopsies in cross-country skiers. Respiration 2000;67(4):417–25.
74. Kaltsatou A, Kouidi E, Fotiou D, et al. The use of pupillometry in the assessment of cardiac autonomic function in elite different type trained athletes. Eur J Appl Physiol 2011;111(9):2079–87.
75. Virchow JC, Backer V, de Blay F, et al. Defining moderate asthma exacerbations in clinical trials based on ATS/ERS joint statement. Respir Med 2015;109(5): 547–56.

Nonpharmacologic Strategies to Manage Exercise-Induced Bronchoconstriction

John Dickinson, PhD[a], Israel Amirav, MD[b],
Morten Hostrup, PhD[c,d,*]

KEYWORDS

- Warm-up • Face mask • Asthma • Pollution • Avoidance • Athletes • Nutrition
- Training

KEY POINTS

- There is emerging evidence that nonpharmacologic strategies can be used to supplement traditional therapy to reduce exercise-induced bronchoconstriction (EIB) severity and lessen respiratory symptoms associated with exercise.
- Most investigations into nonpharmacologic strategies have included nonathletes; extrapolating to athletes should be done with caution, and studies in athletes with EIB are encouraged.
- There is currently insufficient evidence to support the use of any nonpharmacologic EIB treatment strategy in the absence of regular pharmaceutical therapy for EIB.

INTRODUCTION

Exercise-induced bronchoconstriction (EIB) is an asthma-related condition, which occurs during or after exercise as a result of large volumes of unconditioned air entering the lower airways to meet the increased ventilatory demands of exercise.[1,2] In susceptible individuals, EIB arises via multiple mechanisms that may involve dehydration of airway surface liquid, mucosal cooling, and epithelial damage, which induce an airway inflammatory response (involving histamine, neuropeptides, leukotrienes,

Disclosure Statement: Authors have no conflicting interests.
[a] School of Sport and Exercise Sciences, University of Kent, UK; [b] Department of Paediatrics, University of Alberta, Edmonton, Canada; [c] Department of Nutrition, Exercise and Sports, University of Copenhagen, August Krogh 2nd Floor, Universitetsparken 13, Copenhagen DK-2100, Denmark; [d] Department of Respiratory Medicine, Bispebjerg University Hospital, Copenhagen, Denmark
* Corresponding author. Department of Nutrition, Exercise and Sports, University of Copenhagen, August Krogh 2nd Floor, Universitetsparken 13, Copenhagen DK-2100, Denmark.
E-mail address: mhostrup@nexs.ku.dk

Immunol Allergy Clin N Am 38 (2018) 245–258
https://doi.org/10.1016/j.iac.2018.01.012

and prostaglandins) with resultant airway smooth muscle constriction.[3] Management of EIB in athletes is almost exclusively based on pharmacologic therapies (see Vibeke Backer and John Mastronarde's article, "Pharmacologic Strategies for Exercise-Induced Bronchospasm with a Focus on Athletes," in this issue), such as glucocorticoids and β_2-agonists.[1,2] Although clinical data on nonpharmacologic therapies have been equivocal, there is emerging evidence that nonpharmacologic strategies could be used to supplement traditional therapy to reduce EIB severity and lessen exercise respiratory symptoms (Table 1). This article reviews the evidence and provides recommendations for the use of nonpharmacologic strategies in the management of EIB.

PRE-EXERCISE WARM-UP

In approximately half of those who suffer from EIB, high-intensity pre-exercise warm-up effectively protects against subsequent bronchoconstriction.[3] A recent systematic review[54] reported that intermittent high-intensity pre-exercise warm-up (repetitive sprints of approximately 30 s close to peak oxygen consumption or maximum heart rate) provides approximately 10% reduction in the fall in the forced expired volume in the first second of expiration (FEV_1) postexercise, whereas neither low-intensity nor continued high-intensity pre-exercise warm-up provides significant protection in individuals with EIB.

The refractory period or refractory effect that is induced after a first exercise bout has frequency been proposed to explain why high-intensity warm-ups protect against EIB. It has been proposed that the first exercise induces a variable period (called the refractory period) during which (2–4 h) subsequent exercise does not result in EIB. Preceding exercise may deplete constrictive mediators, induce secretion of protective mediators (particularly prostaglandins), and cause desensitization of smooth muscle to bronchoconstrictive mediators.[3] Regardless of the mechanism, there is good evidence to suggest a clinical benefit of warm-ups in protecting against EIB.

Although high-intensity exercise warm-ups may attenuate EIB,[3,54] the exercise intensity that is required for the warm-up may potentially cause perturbations in the exercising musculature and compromise subsequent exercise performance.[4] Emerging evidence suggests, however, that isolated respiratory warm-ups can provide similar bronchoprotective effects as whole-body warm-ups.[55] Instead of using whole-body warm-up, a recent study[55] evaluated the effect of a respiratory-only warm-up on subsequent decline in FEV_1 induced by exhaustive cycling (approximately 14 minutes). In that study, subjects performed normocapnic hyperpnea at different intensities (30%–80% of maximum voluntary ventilation). All hyperpnea sessions attenuated postexercise decline in FEV_1 regardless of the intensity of the hyperpnea session conducted and without compromising cycling performance.[55] Perception of respiratory dyspnea was also reduced by preceding normocapnic hyperpnea. Consequently, both pre-exercise whole-body and respiratory warm-ups may be used to protect against EIB.

AVOIDANCE OF TRIGGERS
Heat and Moisture Exchanger Face Masks

Exercise in dry and cold environments can be a significant trigger of bronchoconstriction. The bronchoconstriction is thought to be caused by dehydration of the airway surface liquid, which causes cell shrinkage and release of inflammatory mediators, precipitating airway smooth muscle constriction.[56] Repeated exposure of the airways to cold dry air may also lead to airway epithelial cell damage, microvascular leakage,

Table 1
Nonpharmacologic strategies to manage exercise-induced bronchoconstriction

Strategy	Intervention	Potential Effect	Evidence Level	Pitfalls	References
Pre-exercise warm-up	Repetitive 30-s bouts close to VO_{2max}/HR_{max}	Reduces postexercise fall in FEV_1	Good	May accumulate peripheral fatigue prior to exertion	3–4
Face masks	HME face masks	Reduces postexercise fall in FEV_1	Insufficient	May affect ventilation and be associated with discomfort	5–8
Omega-3 fatty acid supplementation	3 g/d EPA and 2 g/d DHA	Reduces systemic inflammation Reduces airway inflammation Reduces postexercise fall in FEV_1	Medium Insufficient Insufficient	Side effects: acid reflux, bloating, diarrhea, and nausea	9–13
Caffeine	5–10 mg/kg bw	Induces bronchodilation Reduces postexercise fall in FEV_1 Improves respiratory muscle fatigue resilience Counteracts exercise-induced hypoxemia	Good Medium Medium Insufficient	Slow absorption Side effects: muscle tremors, tachycardia	14–21
Vitamins and antioxidants	1500 mg/d vitamin C 64 mg/d β-carotene	Reduces systemic inflammation Scavenge ROS Reduces postexercise fall in FEV_1	Medium Medium Insufficient	Side effects: diarrhea, vomiting, headache, insomnia, nausea, kidney stones	22–33
Breathing control	See **Table 2**	Reduces perception of respiratory symptoms	Insufficient		34–37
Respiratory muscle training	30 breaths × 2/d at 50% of MIP	Improves respiratory muscle fatigue resilience Reduces asthma severity	Good Insufficient	Time-consuming	38–53

Abbreviations: HR_{max}, maximum heart rate; MIP, maximum inspiratory pressure; ROS, reactive oxygen species; VO_{2max}, maximum oxygen consumption.

and airway remodeling, which may worsen asthma severity.[57] Given the increased risk of bronchoconstriction in dry and cold environments, individuals with asthma may be advised to avoid exercise outside. This places obvious constraints on athletes with asthma-related conditions who have to train and compete in dry and cold environments and also the proportion of individuals with asthma who engage in physical activity as part of their daily routines during the winter months.

Face masks that incorporate a heat and moisture exchanger (HME) are a novel non-pharmacologic tool to counteract EIB in dry and cold environments. Although few studies have investigated the efficacy of HME face masks in counteracting EIB, some studies have demonstrated a protective effect as measured by an attenuation in postexercise decline in FEV_1.[5-8] This suggests that individuals with asthma may use HME face masks to protect against EIB when they engage in moderate to vigorous exercise in cold dry environments. Currently, it is unknown whether the HME face masks reduce airway inflammation over acute and multiple bouts of exercise. Nor is it known whether HME face masks reduce respiratory symptoms and β_2-agonists usage over several weeks of engaging in exercise in dry cold environments. If HME face masks are considered as part of a nonpharmaceutical therapy plan, the design of the masks needs to be considered, because individuals with asthma-related conditions are unlikely to wear the masks if they find the masks large and cumbersome. Athletes may not see HME face masks as a viable strategy to prevent EIB because the masks may not be practical wear to achieve optimal sporting performance or permitted by the rules of the sport.

Air Pollution

Air pollution has been shown to increase asthma severity and may have significant effects on athletes due to the high ventilation rates they achieve and sustain during intense exercise.[58] Air quality is inversely correlated with exercise-induced respiratory symptoms.[59] The risk is also greater in those athletes who train on a regular basis in environments with poor air quality.[60] Small particles, in particular ultrafine ones (<100-nm diameter) like those from combustion engines, have high lung deposition and may cause epithelial damage. These particles include ozone, sulfur dioxide, nitrogen oxides, and particulate matter (PM) (PM smaller than 2.5-μm diameter). Ice skaters are particularly exposed to combination of cold dry air as well as PM less than 1-μm diameter in confined spaces of indoor ice arenas and rom multiple ice-resurfacings by gas-powered or propane-powered machines. Particle inhalations have been shown to induce oxidative stress, airway inflammation, and airway remodeling. All these result in higher prevalence of asthma symptoms and great degree of small airway dysfunction.[61-64]

With regard to management, mechanical barriers, such as face masks, may help reduce the effects of polluted particles.[5] Avoidance of training in low humidity conditions or during times of high levels of atmospheric pollutants is advisable, yet its practical usage and scientific benefit is still questionable. Similarly, whenever possible, it may be recommended to avoid training close to busy major roadways or during rush hours or other times of elevated vehicular congestion.[65]

Swimming

The pathogenic mechanisms of EIB classically involve both osmolar and vascular changes in the airways in addition to cooling of the airways.[2,56] Increased minute ventilation during exercise requires significant warming and humidification of the inspired air. The resulting respiratory heat and water loss from the airway mucosa into the inspired air may release bronchoconstrictive mediators. In that respect, sports in warm humid environments, such as indoor pools, are encouraged. Swimming has often been recommended as a less asthmogenic trigger compared with other sports, because of the humid environment. Yet, a recent Cochrane review concluded that there is insufficient evidence to suggest that aquatic-based exercise is superior to comparative nonaquatic exercise in asthmatics.[66]

Chlorination is the most commonly used method for ensuring water hygiene in swimming pools. Chlorine gas and its aerosol byproducts (eg, trichloramine, hypochlorous acid, and monochloramine and dichloramine), which float just above the water surface, may affect the nose, pharynx, larynx, trachea, and bronchi, with chronic exposure leading to structural epithelial changes. During exercise, nasal breathing at rest shifts to oronasal breathing, thereby significantly reducing the filtering effect of the nose. Aerosol particles travel and deposit further into the lung. Trichloramine gas formed in chlorinated pools was suggested as a cause for EIB in competitive swimmers and increased airway hyperreactivity (as measured by methacholine or eucapnic voluntary hyperventilation [EVH] challenge) has been demonstrated in swimmers.[67–69] Increasing evidence supports the notion that chronic repetitive swimming in indoor pools may induce airway epithelial damage, inflammation, and remodeling[68–70] and increase the risk for atopy and asthma.[71–73] A recent study found increased levels of 8-isoprostane (as a marker of airway oxidative stress) in the exhale breath condensate of competitive swimmers after a swimming session.[72] Whenever possible, swimmers should train in pools cleaned with nonchlorine water disinfection methods (such as copper/silver and ozone) as well as in well-ventilated pool environments. Yet, apart for some case reports,[74] the scientific evidence to support or refute many of these recommendations is lacking.

DIETARY STRATEGIES
Omega-3 Fatty Acid Supplementation

Populations who consume large quantities of oily fish have a lower prevalence of asthma.[75] Oily fish are rich in omega-3 fatty acids: eicosapentaenoic acid (EPA) and docosahexaenoic acid (DHA). EPA and DHA are precursors to powerful agents involved in the resolution of inflammation. Two mechanisms of action underpinning the anti-inflammatory bioactions include the ability of EPA to compete with arachidonic acid as a substrate for cyclooxygenase-2 and 5-lipoxygenase enzymes and be converted to less inflammatory leukotrienes and prostanoids[76,77] and to generate the potent anti-inflammatory E-series resolvins.[76] DHA may also alter gene transcription and translation via direct or indirect actions on intracellular signaling pathways.[78]

The anti-inflammatory properties of EPA and DHA make a diet high in oily fish an attractive addition to the therapy for individuals with EIB. Initial investigations demonstrated 10 weeks' dietary supplementation of EPA, 3.2 g/d, and DHA, 2.2 g/d, reduced leukotriene production by 50% but not reduction in postexercise decline in FEV_1 in asthmatics.[9] Using the same EPA and DHA dietary supplementation over a 3-week period, however, Mickleborough and coworkers[10,11] reported significant reductions in airway inflammation, which was accompanied by 64% to 80% reductions in FEV_1 fall postexercise in individuals with EIB. Postexercise decline in FEV_1, while on EPA and DHA supplementation, was similar to that in the non-EIB control group. In addition, EPA, 3.2 g/d, and DHA, 2 g/d, were observed as favorably as montelukast, 10 mg/d, in reducing airway inflammation and hyperpnea-induced bronchoconstriction in participants with mild to moderate persistent asthma.[12] There seems, however, no additional benefit of combining EPA and DHA supplementation with montelukast, 10 mg.[12] Furthermore, a recent pilot study found no beneficial effect of vitamin D and fish oil supplementation for 3 weeks on reduction in FEV_1 induced by EVH in recreational athletes with EIB.[79]

Recently, the marine lipid fraction of the New Zealand green-lipped mussel (Perna canaliculus), PCSO-524, which is rich in omega-3 fatty acids, has been shown to produce similar reductions in inflammation and bronchoconstriction (57% reduction of FEV_1 fall) after an EVH challenge.[80] In this investigation, the attenuation of airway inflammation and bronchoconstriction cannot be explained entirely by the EPA and DHA content of PCSO-524, because the amounts of EPA and DHA consumed daily were only 72 mg and 48 mg, respectively. Therefore, it may be that the additional constituents of PCSO-524 act synergistically with EPA and DHA to bring about the antiinflammatory effect and reduction in bronchoconstriction.

Although a low intake of EPA and DHA does not seem a safety issue, a few side effects can occur, such as a fishy aftertaste, flatulence, acid reflux, bloating, diarrhea, nausea, and possibly an increased risk of bleeding and immunosuppression with a high intake of omega-3 fatty acids.[13] The initial investigations provide promise for EPA and DHA dietary supplementation to protect against EIB and associated airway inflammation. Large-scale clinical studies in individuals with EIB are required, however, to determine the minimum effective dose and duration required to observe the beneficial effect and to compare the effect of combining omega-3 fatty acid supplementation with prevention inhaler therapy (eg, inhaled glucocorticoids).

Caffeine

Caffeine (1,3,7-trimethylxanthine) is among the most commonly used supplements by athletes.[81] Although formerly subjected to antidoping regulations, the restrictions on caffeine were lifted by the World Anti-Doping Agency in 2004 and it can as such be used freely in and out of competition. Caffeine works as a nonselective competitive adenosine receptor antagonist for all subtypes of the adenosine receptor[82,83] but may also act as a phosphodiesterase inhibitor.[84] Accordingly, caffeine induces intracellular cyclic adenosine monophosphate–dependent/protein kinase A signaling, which like β_2-agonists, causes smooth muscle relaxation.[85] Studies have shown dose-related bronchodilator effects of caffeine on basal airway function.[86] The interest in caffeine as a bronchoprotective agent started approximately 30 years ago when Becker and coworkers[14] observed that 10 mg/kilogram of body weight (kg bw) of orally ingested caffeine had a similar bronchodilating effect as oral theophylline, 5 mg/kg bw, in children with asthma.[14] Comparable bronchodilating effect was later shown in adult asthma patients after ingestion of caffeine,[15] 5 mg/kg bw, or 3 cups of coffee.[16]

Although caffeine shows promise as a bronchodilator, only a few studies have investigated its potential to counteract EIB, none of which has been performed in athletes. In nonathletes, ingestion of caffeine was shown to have a postexercise bronchoprotective effect compared with placebo in individuals with EIB.[17] Although postexercise decline in FEV_1 was 24% for placebo, it was less than 1% after ingestion of caffeine, 7 mg/kg bw, and 8% after caffeine, 3 mg/kg bw. In accordance with this observation, Duffy and Phillips[18] observed that ingestion of caffeine, 10 mg/kg bw, reduced bronchoconstrictor response to EVH-provocation compared with placebo in EVH-positive individuals. When compared with inhalation of β_2-agonist salbutamol (albuterol, 180 mg), ingestion of caffeine, 9 mg/kg bw, was shown as effective as salbutamol in attenuating postexercise reduction in FEV_1 in asthmatics with EIB.[19]

Aside from its bronchoprotective effect, caffeine has a variety of other effects of relevance for airway function during exercise. During submaximal exercise, as little oral caffeine as 3 mg/kg bw has been shown to modulate ventilatory dynamics by reducing the physiologic dead space ventilation/tidal volume ratio and breathing frequency while concurrently increasing tidal volume.[87,88] In addition, caffeine may counteract exercise-induced hypoxemia (desaturation) in elite athletes at submaximal intensities[20] and improve respiratory muscle fatigue resilience.[21]

Despite the small number of studies undertaken, there is some evidence to suggest that caffeine has the potential to reduce EIB severity and improve ventilatory dynamics and respiratory muscle fatigue resilience during exercise. The amount of orally ingested caffeine needed for bronchoprotection is approximately 5 mg/kg bw to 10 mg/kg bw, equivalent to 2 cups to 4 cups of coffee. It seems, however, that the bronchoprotective effect of caffeine is highly individual. A limitation of caffeine is the slow absorption rate when ingested, giving rise to a bronchodilator response 2 hours after ingestion. Future studies should investigate more thoroughly the therapeutic efficacy of caffeine as a bronchoprotective substance during exercise in athletes with EIB.

Vitamins and Antioxidants

Supplementation with various vitamins and antioxidants has attracted some attention as a means to counteract EIB because of their ability to suppress proinflammatory signaling,[22] to lower levels of histamine[23,24] and prostaglandin $F2\alpha$,[25] and to scavenge reactive oxygen species.[26,27] In practical terms, however, interpretation of the therapeutic efficacy of each individual vitamin and antioxidant as bronchoprotective substances in EIB is limited by the small number of studies that have been undertaken in individuals with EIB, especially in athletes. Most convincing is the bronchoprotective effect of acute and chronic supplementation with vitamin C on postexercise decline in FEV_1 in individuals with EIB.[25,28–30] In addition, 1 week supplementation with β-carotene (64 mg), a provitamin A carotenoid, has been shown to reduce postexercise reduction in FEV_1.[31] Conflicting results have been observed after 1-week supplementation with the carotenoid lycopene (30 mg), in which a postexercise bronchoprotective effect was found in asthmatic individuals with EIB, whereas adolescent athletes with EIB had no effect.[32,33]

STRATEGIES TO REDUCE PERCEPTION OF EXERTIONAL DYSPNEA

Strategies that may help control EIB are discussed previously. In addition, there may be a role for using breathing control and inspiratory muscle training (IMT) to enable athletes with EIB to reduce perceptions of exertional dyspnea.

Breathing Control

A significant symptom of EIB is dyspnea during and after exercise. There are a variety of breathing exercises that may benefit individuals who experience asthma/EIB exacerbations that include yogic breathing[34–36] and physiotherapist-supervised breathing training.[37] Although these forms of breathing control exercises may not be able to reduce asthma severity, they may be able to reduce the perception of respiratory symptoms and increase perception of asthma control.[34] Moreover, breathing exercises have been shown to improve quality of life,[35] reduce use of relief medication,[35] and reduce the levels of anxiety and depression[37] and airway hyperresponsiveness.[36] Future research is required to understand the mechanisms behind these observations in asthmatic individuals.

It is currently unknown how these forms of breathing control exercises may be beneficial for athletes with EIB, whose main symptoms are experienced during exercise. The use of breathing training, however, incorporating IMT and breathing technique training (**Table 2**), has been shown helpful in reducing the perception of breathing in an athlete with nonasthmatic exercise respiratory conditions.[38] Future research is required to investigate how athletes with EIB respond to using breathing exercises. Furthermore, the current breathing control methods may need to be adapted to replicate respiratory control during exercise rather than focusing on breathing control at rest.

Respiratory Muscle Training

Respiratory muscle training is an easy and cheap way to enhance both inspiratory and expiratory muscle strength[39] and also has been associated with improvements in exercise performance during various exercise protocols in healthy individuals.[40,41] Despite decades of research into the applications of respiratory muscle training, the area is still controversial and subject to scientific debate.[42–44] Respiratory muscle training has shown some promise in the management of chronic obstructive pulmonary disease,[45] inspiratory stridor,[38] and exercise-induced vocal cord dysfunction.[46,47] Although studies also have shown that respiratory muscle training may have beneficial effects on asthma severity and β_2-agonist usage,[48–50] a recent Cochrane review, based on 113 asthmatics, concluded that there is no conclusive evidence to support or refute the therapeutic efficacy of IMT in asthma.[51] Nevertheless, given individuals with EIB may experience airway obstruction and airflow limitation during intense exercise,[52] which potentially puts a larger work load on respiratory muscles,[3,53] it could be speculated that respiratory muscle training may be beneficial for athletes with EIB. To the authors' knowledge, however, no studies have investigated the effectiveness of respiratory muscle training on EIB severity.[89]

SUMMARY AND FUTURE CONSIDERATIONS

There are numerous nonpharmacologic strategies that can be used to support the treatment of EIB; however, the evidence is inconclusive and future studies are encouraged before any recommendations are implemented. There is currently insufficient

Table 2 Summary of breathing training for athletes	
Breathing Control Methods	**Overview**
Breathing technique	Encourage initiation of inspiration from the lower rib cage. Inspiratory maneuver should be smooth with little tension through the shoulders and neck. Aids, such as elastic strap or hands placed on sides of torso over lower ribs, can be used to help athletes. Athlete can begin to attempt to practice this technique in functional sport specific positions.
IMT	Ensure breathing technique is addressed before initiating IMT. Athletes with poor breathing technique, who proceed directly to IMT, may experience exacerbation of their symptoms. IMT should incorporate forceful inspiratory maneuvers through a handheld device providing resistance to the inspired airflow. Focus during the IMT should be on good breathing technique (as described previously). An IMT session should comprise 30 continuous forced inspiratory efforts at the equivalent of 30 breath repetitions maximum, with relaxed expiration.

Data from Dickinson J, McConnell A, Ross E, et al. The BASES expert statement on assessment and management of non-asthma related breathing problems in athletes. The Sport and Exercise Scientist, Issue 45, Autumn 2015, British Association of Sport and Exercise Sciences, www.bases.org.uk.

evidence to support the use of any nonpharmacologic EIB treatment strategy in the absence of regular pharmaceutical therapy for EIB. Although there are some encouraging findings with regard to nutritional supplementation and respiratory muscle training, future studies are encouraged, especially in athletes. Most studies have included nonathletes and extrapolation to athletes should, therefore, be done with caution. Furthermore, data on other commonly used supplements by athletes, such as β-alanine and creatine, are lacking in relation to EIB. For instance, β-alanine supplementation increases intracellular content of carnosine, which, among other factors,[90] may affect nitric oxide production and modulate inflammation,[91,92] both of which could affect EIB severity. In addition, creatine supplementation has been shown to exacerbate airway inflammation, increase airway hyperresponsiveness, and induce smooth muscle thickening in mice.[93] No studies, however, have, to the authors' knowledge, investigated the effect of creatine supplementation on EIB severity in athletes. Consequently, there are numerous nonpharmacologic strategies yet to be studied in athletes with EIB.

REFERENCES

1. Fitch KD, Sue-Chu M, Anderson SD, et al. Asthma and the elite athlete: summary of the International Olympic Committee's consensus conference, Lausanne, Switzerland, January 22-24, 2008. J Allergy Clin Immunol 2008;122(2):254–60.
2. Price OJ, Hull JH, Backer V, et al. The impact of exercise-induced bronchoconstriction on athletic performance: a systematic review. Sports Med 2014;44(12): 1749–61.
3. Larsson J, Anderson SD, Dahlén SE, et al. Refractoriness to exercise challenge: a review of the mechanisms old and new. Immunol Allergy Clin North Am 2013; 33(3):329–35.
4. Hostrup M, Bangsbo J. Limitations in intense exercise performance of athletes - effect of speed endurance training on ion handling and fatigue development. J Physiol 2017;595(9):2897–913.
5. Beuther DA, Martin RJ. Efficacy of a heat exchanger mask in cold exercise-induced asthma. Chest 2006;129(5):1188–93.
6. Brenner A, Weiser P, Krogh L, et al. Effectiveness of a portable face mask in attenuating exercise-induced asthma. JAMA 1980;244:2196–8.
7. Millqvist E, Bengtsson U, Löwhagen O. Combining a beta2-agonist with a face mask to prevent exercise-induced bronchoconstriction. Allergy 2000;55:672–5.
8. Nisar M, Spence D, West D, et al. A mask to modify inspired air temperature and humidity and its effect on exercise induced asthma. Thorax 1992;47:446–50.
9. Arm JP, Horton CE, Mencia-Huerta JM, et al. Effect of dietary supplementation with fish oil lipids on mild asthma. Thorax 1988;43(2):84–92.
10. Mickleborough TD, Murray RL, Ionescu AA, et al. Fish oil supplementation reduces severity of exercise-induced bronchoconstriction in elite athletes. Am J Respir Crit Care Med 2003;168(10):1181–9.
11. Mickleborough TD, Lindley MR, Ionescu AA, et al. Protective effect of fish oil supplementation on exercise-induced bronchoconstriction in asthma. Chest 2006; 129(1):39–49.
12. Tecklenburg-Lund S, Mickleborough TD, Turner LA, et al. Randomized controlled trial of fish oil and montelukast and their combination on airway inflammation and hyperpnea-induced bronchoconstriction. PLoS One 2010;5(10):e13487.
13. Mickleborough TD, Lindley MR. Omega-3 fatty acids: a potential future treatment for asthma? Expert Rev Respir Med 2013;7(6):577–80.

14. Becker AB, Simons KJ, Gillespie CA, et al. The bronchodilator effects and pharmacokinetics of caffeine in asthma. N Eng J Med 1984;310:743–6.
15. Bukowskyj M, Nakatsu K. The bronchodilator effect of caffeine in adult asthmatics. Am Rev Respir Dis 1987;135(1):173–5.
16. Gong H Jr, Simmons MS, Tashkin DP, et al. Bronchodilator effects of caffeine in coffee. Chest 1986;89:335–42.
17. Kivity S, Ben Aharon Y, Man A, et al. The effect of caffeine on exercise-induced bronchoconstriction. Chest 1990;97(5):1083–5.
18. Duffy P, Phillips YY. Caffeine consumption decreases the response to bronchoprovocation challenge with dry gas hyperventilation. Chest 1991;99(6):1374–7.
19. VanHaitsma TA, Mickleborough T, Stager JM, et al. Comparative effects of caffeine and albuterol on the bronchoconstrictor response to exercise in asthmatic athletes. Int J Sports Med 2010;31(4):231–6.
20. Chapman RF, Stager JM. Caffeine stimulates ventilation in athletes with exercise-induced hypoxemia. Med Sci Sports Exerc 2008;40(6):1080–6.
21. Supinski GS, Levin S, Kelsen SG. Caffeine effect on respiratory muscle endurance and sense of effort during loaded breathing. J Appl Physiol 1986;60(6):2040–7.
22. Jiang Q. Natural forms of vitamin E: metabolism, antioxidant, and anti-inflammatory activities and their role in disease prevention and therapy. Free Radic Biol Med 2014;72:76–90.
23. Johnston CS, Retrum KR, Srilakshmi JC. Antihistamine effects and complications of supplemental vitamin C. J Am Diet Assoc 1992;92(8):988–9.
24. Johnston CS, Solomon RE, Corte C. Vitamin C depletion is associated with alterations in blood histamine and plasma free carnitine in adults. J Am Coll Nutr 1996;15(6):586–91.
25. Tecklenburg SL, Mickleborough TD, Fly AD, et al. Ascorbic acid supplementation attenuates exercise-induced bronchoconstriction in patients with asthma. Respir Med 2007;101(8):1770–8.
26. Traber MG, Stevens JF. Vitamins C and E: beneficial effects from a mechanistic perspective. Free Radic Biol Med 2011;51(5):1000–13.
27. Ashton T, Young IS, Peters JR, et al. Electron spin resonance spectroscopy, exercise, and oxidative stress: an ascorbic acid intervention study. J Appl Physiol 1999;87(6):2032–6.
28. Schachter EN, Schlesinger A. The attenuation of exercise-induced bronchospasm by ascorbic acid. Ann Allergy 1982;49(3):146–51.
29. Cohen HA, Neuman I, Nahum H. Blocking effect of vitamin C in exercise-induced asthma. Arch Pediatr Adolesc Med 1997;151(4):367–70.
30. Hemilä H. The effect of vitamin C on bronchoconstriction and respiratory symptoms caused by exercise: a review and statistical analysis. Allergy Asthma Clin Immunol 2014;10(1):58.
31. Neuman I, Nahum H, Ben-Amotz A. Prevention of exercise-induced asthma by a natural isomer mixture of beta-carotene. Ann Allergy Asthma Immunol 1999;82(6):549–53.
32. Neuman I, Nahum H, Ben-Amotz A. Reduction of exercise-induced asthma oxidative stress by lycopene, a natural antioxidant. Allergy 2000;55(12):1184–9.
33. Falk B, Gorev R, Zigel L, et al. Effect of lycopene supplementation on lung function after exercise in young athletes who complain of exercise-induced bronchoconstriction symptoms. Ann Allergy Asthma Immunol 2005;94(4):480–5.
34. Karam M, Kaur B, Baptist A. A modified breathing exercise program for asthma is easy to perform and effective. J Asthma 2017;54(2):217–22.

35. Vempati R, Bijlani RL, Deepak KK. The efficacy of a comprehensive lifestyle modification programme based on yoga in the management of bronchial asthma: a randomized controlled trial. BMC Pulm Med 2009;9:37.

36. Manocha R, Marks G, Kenchington P, et al. Sahaja yoga in the management of moderate to severe asthma: a randomised controlled trial. Thorax 2002;57(2): 110–5.

37. Thomas M, McKinley RK, Mellor S, et al. Breathing exercises for asthma: a randomised controlled trial. Thorax 2009;64(1):55–61.

38. Dickinson J, Whyte G, McConnell A. Inspiratory muscle training: a simple cost-effective treatment for inspiratory stridor. Br J Sports Med 2007;41(10):694–5.

39. Romer LM, McConnell AK. Specificity and reversibility of inspiratory muscle training. Med Sci Sports Exerc 2003;35(2):237–44.

40. Kilding AE, Brown S, McConnell AK. Inspiratory muscle training improves 100 and 200 m swimming performance. Eur J Appl Physiol 2010;108(3):505–11.

41. Illi SK, Held U, Frank I, et al. Effect of respiratory muscle training on exercise performance in healthy individuals: a systematic review and meta-analysis. Sports Med 2012;42(8):707–24.

42. McConnell AK. CrossTalk opposing view: respiratory muscle training does improve exercise tolerance. J Physiol 2012;590(15):3397–8.

43. Mickleborough TD, Stager JM, Chatham K, et al. Pulmonary adaptations to swim and inspiratory muscle training. Eur J Appl Physiol 2008;103(6):635–46.

44. Patel MS, Hart N, Polkey MI. CrossTalk proposal: training the respiratory muscles does not improve exercise tolerance. J Physiol 2012;590(15):3393–5.

45. Geddes EL, O'Brien K, Reid WD, et al. Inspiratory muscle training in adults with chronic obstructive pulmonary disease: an update of a systematic review. Respir Med 2008;102(12):1715–29.

46. Mathers-Schmidt BA, Brilla LR. Inspiratory muscle training in exercise-induced paradoxical vocal fold motion. J Voice 2005;19(4):635–44.

47. Ruddy BH, Davenport P, Baylor J, et al. Inspiratory muscle strength training with behavioral therapy in a case of a rower with presumed exercise-induced paradoxical vocal-fold dysfunction. Int J Pediatr Otorhinolaryngol 2004;68(10): 1327–32.

48. Turner LA, Mickleborough TD, McConnell AK, et al. Effect of inspiratory muscle training on exercise tolerance in asthmatic individuals. Med Sci Sports Exerc 2011;43(11):2031–8.

49. Weiner P, Azgad Y, Ganam R, et al. Inspiratory muscle training in patients with bronchial asthma. Chest 1992;102(5):1357–61.

50. Weiner P, Berar-Yanay N, Davidovich A, et al. Specific inspiratory muscle training in patients with mild asthma with high consumption of inhaled beta(2)-agonists. Chest 2000;117(3):722–7.

51. Silva IS, Fregonezi GA, Dias FA, et al. Inspiratory muscle training for asthma. Cochrane Database Syst Rev 2013;(9):CD003792.

52. Johnson BD, Scanlon PD, Beck KC. Regulation of ventilatory capacity during exercise in asthmatics. J Appl Physiol 1995;79(3):892–901.

53. Kosmas EN, Milic-Emili J, Polychronaki A, et al. Exercise-induced flow limitation, dynamic hyperinflation and exercise capacity in patients with bronchial asthma. Eur Respir J 2004;24(3):378–84.

54. Stickland MK, Rowe BH, Spooner CH, et al. Effect of warm-up exercise on exercise-induced bronchoconstriction. Med Sci Sports Exerc 2012;44(3):383–91.

55. Eichenberger PA, Scherer TA, Spengler CM. Pre-exercise hyperpnea attenuates exercise-induced bronchoconstriction without affecting performance. PLoS One 2016;11(11):e0167318.
56. Anderson SD, Kippelen P. Airway injury as a mechanism for exercise-induced bronchoconstriction in elite athletes. J Allergy Clin Immunol 2008;122(2):225–35.
57. Karjalainen E, Laitinen A, Sue-Chu M, et al. Evidence of airway inflammation and remodeling in ski athletes with and without bronchial hyperresponsiveness to methacholine. Am J Respir Crit Care Med 2000;161:2086–91.
58. Guarnieri M, Balmes J. Outdoor air pollution and asthma. Lancet 2014;383: 1581–92.
59. Rundell KW, Spiering BA, Judelson DA, et al. Bronchoconstriction during cross-country skiing: is there really a refractory period? Med Sci Sports Exerc 2003; 35(1):18–26.
60. Bernard A, Nickmilder M, Voisin C. Outdoor swimming pools and the risks of asthma and allergies during adolescence. Eur Respir J 2008;32(4):979–88.
61. Lumme A, Haahtela T, Ounap J, et al. Airway inflammation, bronchial hyperresponsiveness and asthma in elite ice hockey players. Eur Respir J 2003;22(1): 113–7.
62. Rundell KW, Spiering BA, Evans TM, et al. Baseline lung function, exercise-induced bronchoconstriction, and asthma-like symptoms in elite women ice hockey players. Med Sci Sports Exerc 2004;36(3):405–10.
63. Rundell KW, Im J, Mayers LB, et al. Self-reported symptoms and exercise-induced asthma in the elite athlete. Med Sci Sports Exerc 2001;33(2):208–13.
64. Rundell KW, Caviston R, Hollenbach AM, et al. Vehicular air pollution, playgrounds, and youth athletic fields. Inhal Toxicol 2006;18(8):541–7.
65. Cutrufello PT, Smoliga JM, Rundell KW. Small things make a big difference: particulate matter and exercise. Sports Med 2012;42(12):1041–58.
66. Silva GAJ, Andriolo BNG, Riera R, et al. Water-based exercise for adults with asthma (review). Cochrane Database Syst Rev 2014;(7):CD003316.
67. Levai IK, Hull JH, Loosemore M, et al. Environmental influence on the prevalence and pattern of airway dysfunction in elite athletes. Respirology 2016;21(8): 1391–6.
68. Bougault V, Boulet LP. Is there a potential link between indoor chlorinated pool environment and airway remodeling/inflammation in swimmers? Expert Rev Respir Med 2012;6(5):469–71.
69. Bougault V, Loubaki L, Joubert P, et al. Airway remodeling and inflammation in competitive swimmers training in indoor chlorinated swimming pools. J Allergy Clin Immunol 2012;129(2):351–8.
70. Sue-Chu M. Winter sports athletes: long-term effects of cold air exposure. Br J Sports Med 2012;46(6):397–401.
71. Bernard A, Carbonnelle S, de Burbure C, et al. Chlorinated pool attendance, atopy, and the risk of asthma during childhood. Environ Health Perspect 2006; 114(10):1567–73.
72. Bernard A, Carbonnelle S, Michel O, et al. Lung hyperpermeability and asthma prevalence in schoolchildren: unexpected associations with the attendance at indoor chlorinated swimming pools. Occup Environ Med 2003;60(6):385–94.
73. Morissette MC, Murray N, Turmel J, et al. Increased exhaled breath condensate 8-isoprostane after a swimming session in competitive swimmers. Eur J Sport Sci 2016;16(5):569–76.
74. Beretta S, Vivaldo T, Morelli M, et al. Swimming pool-induced asthma. J Investig Allergol Clin Immunol 2011;21(3):240–1.

75. Horrobin D. Low prevalences of coronary heart disease (CHD), psoriasis, asthma and rheumatoid arthritis in Eskimos: are they caused by high dietary intake of eicosapentaenoic acid (EPA), a genetic variation of essential fatty acid (EFA) metabolism or a combination of both? Med Hypotheses 1987; 22(4):421–8.

76. Thien F, Hallsworth M, Soh C, et al. Effects of exogenous eicosapentaenoic acid on generation of leukotriene C4 and leukotriene C5 by calcium ionophore-activated human eosinophils in vitro. J Immunol 1993;150:3546–52.

77. Serhan CN, Yang R, Martinod K, et al. Maresins: novel macrophage mediators with potent antiinflammatory and proresolving actions. J Exp Med 2009;206(1): 15–23.

78. Weldon S, Mullen A, Loscher C, et al. Docosahexaenoic acid induces an anti-inflammatory profile in lipopolysaccharide-stimulated human THP-1 macro-phages more effectively than eicosapentaenoic acid. J Nutr Biochem 2007; 18(4):250–8.

79. Price OJ, Hull JH, Howatson G, et al. Vitamin D and omega-3 polyunsaturated fatty acid supplementation in athletes with exercise-induced bronchoconstriction: a pilot study. Expert Rev Respir Med 2015;9(3):369–78.

80. Mickleborough TD, Vaughn CL, Shei RJ, et al. Marine lipid fraction PCSO-524 (lyprinol/omega XL) of the New Zealand green lipped mussel attenuates hyperpnea-induced bronchoconstriction in asthma. Respir Med 2013;107(8): 1152–63.

81. Del Coso J, Muñoz G, Muñoz-Guerra J. Prevalence of caffeine use in elite ath-letes following its removal from the World Anti-Doping Agency list of banned sub-stances. Appl Physiol Nutr Metab 2011;36(4):555–61.

82. Evoniuk G, Jacobson KA, Shamim MT, et al. A1- and A2-selective adenosine an-tagonists: in vivo characterization of cardiovascular effects. J Pharmacol Exp Ther 1987;242(3):882–7.

83. Snyder SH, Katims JJ, Annau Z, et al. Adenosine receptors and behavioral ac-tions of methylxanthines. Proc Natl Acad Sci U S A 1981;78(5):3260–4.

84. Rivedal E, Sanner T. Caffeine and other phosphodiesterase inhibitors are potent inhibitors of the promotional effect of TPA on morphological transformation of hamster embryo cells. Cancer Lett 1985;28(1):9–17.

85. Niewoehner DE, Campe H, Duane S, et al. Mechanisms of airway smooth muscle response to isoproterenol and theophylline. J Appl Physiol Respir Environ Exerc Physiol 1979;47(2):330–6.

86. Welsh EJ, Bara A, Barley E, et al. Caffeine for asthma. Cochrane Database Syst Rev 2010;(1):CD001112.

87. Birnbaum LJ, Herbst JD. Physiologic effects of caffeine on cross-country runners. J Strength Cond Res 2004;18(3):463–5.

88. Brown DD, Knowlton RG, Sullivan JJ, et al. Effect of caffeine ingestion on alveolar ventilation during moderate exercise. Aviat Space Environ Med 1991;62(9 Pt 1): 860–4.

89. Shei RJ, Paris HL, Wilhite DP, et al. The role of inspiratory muscle training in the management of asthma and exercise-induced bronchoconstriction. Phys Sportsmed 2016;44(4):327–34.

90. Hostrup M, Bangsbo J. Improving beta-alanine supplementation strategy to enhance exercise performance in athletes. J Physiol 2016;594(17):4701–2.

91. Severina IS, Bussygina OG, Pyatakova NV. Carnosine as a regulator of soluble guanylate cyclase. Biochemistry (Mosc) 2000;65(7):783–8.

92. Caruso G, Fresta CG, Martinez-Becerra F, et al. Carnosine modulates nitric oxide in stimulated murine RAW 264.7 macrophages. Mol Cell Biochem 2017;431(1–2): 197–210.

93. Vieira RP, Duarte AC, Claudino RC, et al. Creatine supplementation exacerbates allergic lung inflammation and airway remodeling in mice. Am J Respir Cell Mol Biol 2007;37(6):660–7.

Exercise and Sinonasal Disease

Brecht Steelant, PhD[a], Valerie Hox, MD, PhD[b], Peter W. Hellings, MD, PhD[a,c],
Dominique M. Bullens, MD, PhD[d,e], Sven F. Seys, PhD[a,*]

KEYWORDS

- Rhinitis • Chronic rhinosinusitis • Nasal hyperreactivity • Nasal obstruction
- Exercise-induced rhinitis • Upper airway disease

KEY POINTS

- Rhinitis is more common in athletes compared with the general population.
- Timely and proper treatment of upper airway disease in athletes is likely to positively impact their athletic performance.
- More research is needed to elucidate the mechanisms behind upper airway symptoms in athletes.

INTRODUCTION

Regular physical activity at moderate intensity is beneficial for health and is endorsed by the World Health Organization (WHO).[1] The nose plays a pivotal role in respiratory physiology, as inhaled air is humidified, heated, and filtered in the nose.[2] Impaired nasal function due to allergen-, pathogen- or irritant-induced upper airway disease negatively affects exercise performance.[3] Therefore, the nose and sino-nasal cavities need to function optimally during sport.[4,5]

Rhinitis, defined as symptomatic inflammation of the nasal mucosa causing at least 2 symptoms (congestion, rhinorrhea, nasal pruritis, and/or sneezing), can be caused

Disclosure Statement: The authors declare that they have no competing interests related to this article.
[a] Laboratory of Clinical Immunology, Department of Microbiology and Immunology, KU Leuven, Herestraat 49, Box 811, Leuven 3000, Belgium; [b] Division of Otorhinolaryngology, Cliniques Universitaires Saint-Luc, Hippocrateslaan 10, 1200 Sint-Lambrechts-Woluwe, Brussels, Belgium; [c] Clinical Department of Otorhinolaryngology, Head and Neck Surgery, University Hospitals Leuven, UZ Leuven, Kapucijnevoer 33, Leuven 3000, Belgium; [d] Paediatric Immunology, Department of Microbiology and Immunology, KU Leuven, Herestraat 49, Box 811, Leuven 3000, Belgium; [e] Clinical Department of Pediatrics, University Hospitals Leuven, Herestraat 49, Box 811, Leuven 3000, Belgium
* Corresponding author. Laboratory of Clinical Immunology, Department of Microbiology and Immunology, KU Leuven, Herestraat 49, Box 811, Leuven 3000, Belgium.
E-mail address: sven.seys@kuleuven.be

by infectious organisms, allergic inflammation, or other noninfectious, nonallergic triggers.[6] It occurs in about 30% of the Western population and causes notable impacts on quality of life.[7,8] Rhinosinusitis, inflammation of the nasal mucosa extending to the mucosa of the paranasal sinuses, affects approximately 10% of the general population.[9] It is characterized by 2 or more of the following symptoms: nasal blockage, rhinorrhea, facial pain, and/or smell reduction.[10] Different environmental factors, such as allergens, pathogens and irritants, are known to contribute to the development of sino-nasal disease.[11] Additional factors, including genetic susceptibility and sensitivity of the airway epithelium, are hypothesized to contribute.

It is possible that there are important mechanistic and clinical links between exercise and sino-nasal function. Although the nasal airway contributes for only 10% to the overall minute ventilation at maximal exercise,[12] sino-nasal health may impact the athlete during or outside of exercise. Increased ventilation rates present during exercise increase exposure to allergens, irritants, and pollutants, which subsequently may lead to epithelial cell injury as seen in the development of exercise-induced bronchoconstriction and asthma.[13,14] Indeed, regular intensive physical exercise is considered to be a risk factor for developing asthma and/or exercise-induced bronchoconstriction.[15,16] A limited number of studies have investigated whether intensive exercise on a regular basis by competitive athletes is associated with a higher prevalence of upper respiratory tract diseases, such as rhinitis and rhinosinusitis.[16,17]

In this review, the authors discuss the epidemiology, mechanism, diagnostic approach, and therapies for sino-nasal disease in the athlete as part of a series of articles designed to give a comprehensive review of the treatment of all airways during exercise.

PREVALENCE OF SINO-NASAL DISEASE IN ATHLETES AND DISEASE SUBTYPES

Several studies, with variability in diagnostic criteria for rhinitis as well as variability in specific sports studied, have investigated the prevalence of rhinitis in athletes. These estimates range from 8% to 41%.[18] One study, investigating almost 300 German elite athletes, demonstrated significantly higher rates of rhinitis in athletes compared with the general population (25.4% vs 16.9%).[19] Other large-scale studies in Australian,[20] Italian,[11] and Finnish[21] Olympic athletes provide similar prevalence estimates. A study in US Olympic athletes demonstrated lower rhinitis rates, with only 18% of athletes affected and no difference compared with controls.[22]

The etiologic subtypes of rhinitis can be divided into infectious, allergic, and nonallergic noninfectious rhinitis.

Infectious Rhinitis in Athletes

Viral rhinitis or the common cold is a common illness in humans worldwide. It is generally a mild disease; but in athletes, upper respiratory tract infections (URTIs) represent an enormous burden. They occur at an increased frequency when compared with the general population.[16,17] They are the most common reason for presenting to a sports medicine clinic[17,23] and are the most common medical problem encountered at both winter and summer Olympics.[24,25] For example, during the Sydney 2000 Olympic Games, 33% of all consultations of the New Zealand medical team were categorized as upper respiratory tract illnesses.[25] Clinical studies show a significant increase in the risk to develop a URTI following extreme endurance events, compared with recreational exercise.[26,27] Nieman and colleagues[26] reported that 12.9% of Los Angeles Marathon runners had a URTI in the week following the marathon versus 2.2% of runners who did not participate. Peters and colleagues[27] obtained similar results showing a doubling in prevalence of URTI in runners compared with controls, with the highest prevalence in those who achieved the fastest race times.

Most of these data have been based on self-reported symptoms and have often not been validated with objective measures of infection. Moreover, studies looking for pathogens or infectious parameters have failed to identify an infectious cause in as many as 70% of athletes reporting URTI symptoms.[17,28] This finding suggests that the noninfectious causes of upper airway symptoms may be underestimated in this population.

Allergic Rhinitis in Athletes

The most common cause of chronic rhinitis in the general population is allergy with 23% to 30% affected in Europe and 12% to 30% affected in the United States.[29] Generally, the prevalence of allergic rhinitis is the highest in the adolescent and young adult population,[29] the age range comprising most elite athletes.

Pollen allergy may be particularly problematic for the outdoor athlete. Helenius and colleagues[30] showed in a survey of 49 summer athletes that a clinical presentation of pollen allergy, defined as positive skin prick testing (SPT) in combination with symptoms of seasonal allergic rhinitis, was more common in athletes than in nonathletes. Another study investigating 214 Australian Olympic athletes demonstrated that 41% of the athletes showed a positive SPT response to any one allergen and 29% had a clinically proven seasonal allergic rhinoconjunctivitis.[31] In another series of 265 athletes selected for the Sydney Olympic Games, the prevalence of positive SPT was 32% and 25% of athletes had clinical rhinitis.[32] A questionnaire-based study from Katelaris and colleagues[31] demonstrated a lower quality of life in pollen-allergic athletes, which improved as the pollen count declined.

Nonallergic/Noninfectious Rhinitis and Exercise-Induced Rhinitis in Athletes

Many athletes presumably have nonallergic, noninfectious rhinitis (NANIR) or nonallergic rhinitis (NAR) based on population data,[33] although the specific prevalence data for athletes are not currently available. A recent study investigating field hockey players found lower Allergic Questionnaire for Athletes (AQUA) scores in elite players with rhinitis compared with nonelite players and controls with rhinitis, thus, suggesting (without immunoglobulin E [IgE] detection methods) a nonallergic cause of the upper airway symptoms in the highly trained group.[34] The causal factors hypothesized to induce NANIR symptoms include chemical irritants (chlorination products, ozone, and other indoor or outdoor pollutants) or physical triggers (changes in temperature, humidity, or osmolality). These triggers are typically known to induce symptoms in patients presenting with nasal hyperreactivity (NHR),[35] a disease characteristic that can be present in allergic, infectious, and NANIR.[36]

Some specific sports seem to increase the risk for NAR, including winter sports (likely due to continuous exposure to cold dry air) and swimming (likely due to chronic exposure to chlorine and chlorination byproducts). Bonadonna and colleagues[37] reported a prevalence of almost 50% of cold-induced rhinitis in 144 skiers. This type of rhinitis mainly presented as rhinorrhea and was present in both atopic as well as nonatopic athletes. A study from 2004 showed a significantly decreased baseline nasal patency and mucociliary clearance time in skiers compared with control values.[38] Elite swimmers' airways seem to be particularly affected by the chlorination products used to disinfect swimming pools,[39] and up to 74% of them complain about rhinitis symptoms.[40–42] Some studies suggest a higher prevalence of allergic upper airway inflammation in this athlete population.[42,43] However, it is thought that a substantial part of the swimmers with rhinitis have NAR.[40]

Rhinosinusitis in Athletes

To the authors' knowledge, the prevalence of rhinosinusitis in athletes is largely unknown. The only study reporting on rhinosinusitis prevalence in athletes is the study of swimmers from Gelardi and colleagues,[40] reporting that 3.2% of symptomatic swimmers had rhinosinusitis.[40] Another study describes rhinosinusitis in divers due to barotrauma.[44] Because infectious and allergic rhinitis are considered to be risk factors for the development of rhinosinusitis,[9] it is indeed likely that athletes are also more affected compared with their nonathletic peers.

MECHANISMS LEADING TO EXERCISE-INDUCED RHINITIS

Although few studies investigating the pathophysiology of exercise-induced rhinitis are available, epithelial shedding, neutrophilic pathways, and decreased mucociliary clearance are thought to be involved. Increased sputum neutrophils have been demonstrated in elite swimmers and were associated with the number of training hours.[14,45] Gelardi and colleagues[40] found that, in 43 swimmers with rhinitis, 76% had NAR, of whom 35% showed a neutrophilic type of nasal inflammation. Interestingly, this neutrophilic inflammation in the nonallergic group disappeared after 1 month when swimmers started using a nasal clip. In another study involving 35 elite swimmers, it was found that in all of them the mucociliary transport time was higher than in normal controls.[38] Both studies suggest a direct irritant effect on the airway mucosa and mirror earlier studies showing increased numbers of neutrophils in nasal fluid and reduced nasal mucociliary clearance after a marathon.[46,47] More recently, impaired mucociliary clearance was also shown in healthy athletes after 45-minute runs for 5 days in the polluted streets of Sao Paulo compared with urban forest runs where there was less air pollution.[48] Whether strenuous exercise contributes to the development of allergic sensitization and inflammation remains debated. Some immunologic studies in athletes have suggested a potential shift of the T-lymphocyte population toward a T-helper 2 subtype on excessive exercise, predisposing them to allergic sensitization.[49,50]

Although some athletes experience improvement in nasal function with exercise (through an increase in nasal sympathetic tone),[51] it is thought that the increased ventilation during intensive exercise can induce epithelial injury as well as physical and immunologic changes.[52] In addition, different irritant environments, such as polluted, chlorine-rich, or cold air, might add up or be responsible for these effects as well. Chlorine gas, chloramines (mainly at indoor pools), and hypochlorite may contribute to irritant effects in swimmers.[53] Increased epithelial shedding and release of damage-associated molecular pattern molecules (uric acid and high mobility group box-1) in sputum was demonstrated in cold-air athletes and elite swimmers, respectively.[45] These changes might be responsible for the increased nasal symptoms seen in elite athletes.[54]

DIAGNOSIS OF SINO-NASAL DISEASE IN ATHLETES

Because nasal health is clearly of key importance to the athlete's performance and rhinitis is often underdiagnosed (and undertreated) in this population, early and correct diagnosis of upper airway disease is important.

A thorough history is the cornerstone for making the correct diagnosis. Identification of the symptom-inducing trigger (eg, allergen, infection, cold air, swimming pool, or exercise itself) can give clear indications of the type of airway disease one is dealing with and, thus, an outline for an adequate treatment strategy.

Anterior rhinoscopy is the first-line clinical examination to evaluate the nasal mucosa, to check for signs of infection, and to exclude significant structural abnormalities, such as septal deviation.[55] Nasal endoscopy, on the other hand, offers the advantage of a global evaluation of the nasal cavity and should be considered on suspicion of rhinosinusitis with or without an additional computed tomography scan of the sino-nasal area.[9]

Every athlete presenting with airway symptoms should be screened for allergies as a causal factor of rhinitis. The formal diagnosis of allergic rhinitis is based on a concordance between a typical history of allergic rhinitis symptoms on exposure to the allergen and the detection of allergen-specific IgEs, either by SPT or in the serum by immune assay.[29] The validated AQUA is often used as a screening tool to identify athletes with allergic disease, and a score of greater than 5 has a positive predictive value of 0.94.[56]

When athletes complain about nasal obstruction, several technical examination methods are available to determine nasal patency, including rhinomanometry, acoustic rhinometry, and peak nasal inspiratory flow measurements.[55]

Finally, in selected cases, it might be useful to test for NHR. Several methods have been evaluated to diagnose this condition, but a nasal cold, dry air challenge has been proven to be the most specific and well tolerated and, therefore, is the method of choice.[35] When athletes are specifically presenting with exercise-induced rhinitis, testing for NHR is useful as well as an exercise challenge test, including measurements of nasal obstruction and/or evaluation of nasal secretions before and after exercise. At the current time, exercise challenge tests are not validated or standardized as diagnostic tools for exercise-induced rhinitis.

TREATMENT OF SINO-NASAL DISEASE IN ATHLETES

Elite athletes frequently present with sino-nasal symptoms, which may negatively impact athletic performance and/or recovery.[57,58] The choice of treatment may depend on the severity of the symptoms and the initiating trigger responsible for the symptoms. Additionally, in order to remain in compliance with World Anti-Doping Agency (WADA) mandates, athletes with sino-nasal problems and treating providers must be cognizant of several medications which require therapeutic use exemptions[59] (Table 1). It is, therefore, of utmost importance that athletes with upper airway diseases are provided with recommendations tailored to meet their specific needs.

Avoidance of Environmental Triggers

Intensive exercise in unfavorable environments, such as chlorinated swimming pools, cold air, or areas with high levels of allergens, can lead to an increase in upper respiratory symptoms in specific athletes. Accordingly, avoidance of allergens and/or irritants should be the first step in the treatment of athletes with respiratory diseases. In reality, environmental control is difficult to implement in most cases, especially for athletes participating in sports that occur outdoors in cold weather.

Exposure to irritants, such as chlorine byproducts, should be kept as low as possible. National regulations defining maximum chlorine byproduct levels in swimming pools vary among different countries. The WHO's recent regulations defined a target maximum trichloramine concentration of 0.5 mg/m^3 in the air of indoor swimming pools.[60] Significant ocular and respiratory symptoms have been reported to occur in swimming pool workers and competitive swimmers when airborne

Table 1
Treatment options for sino-nasal diseases in athletes

Treatment	Disease	Side Effects	WADA's Regulations	Annotations/ Comments
Antihistamines	AR	First-generation: sedation, impair reaction time and performance	Currently permitted	Newest molecules: no sedative effect and no liver metabolism
Mast cell stabilizers	AR	—	Currently permitted	Needs to be taken over few days before exposure to obtain symptom control
Antileukotrienes	AR	—	Currently permitted	—
Intranasal steroids	AR, ARS, CRS	Epistaxis, irritation of throat and nose, nasal dryness	Currently permitted	No systemic effects compared with oral/intravenous steroids
Oral/intravenous steroids	AR, ARS, CRS	Multiple	Currently requires therapeutic use exemption	—
Decongestants	AR, ARS, CRS	Elevated heart rate and blood pressure, tremor	Varies based on medication with some medications currently requiring therapeutic use exemption	Rebound effect: nasal congestion worsens
Immunotherapy	AR	Discomfort at site of injection; anaphylaxis	Currently permitted	No exercise in the hours after administration
Antibiotics	ARS, CRS	Varies based on medication	Currently permitted	Choice depends on causative infectious agents

Abbreviations: AR, allergic rhinitis; ARS, acute rhinosinusitis; CRS, chronic rhinosinusitis.
Data from Refs.[73,75,76]

trichloramine levels exceeded 0.5 mg/m^3.[61,62] Regular monitoring of the airborne trichloramine levels might be considered in addition to the daily water analysis in indoor swimming pools.

When avoidance of environmental triggers does not bring sufficient symptom relief, appropriate pharmacotherapy is recommended to treat upper airway symptoms related to exercise.

Antihistamines and Mast Cell Stabilizers

Antihistamines are a first-line treatment of athletes with allergic rhinitis to reduce nasal symptoms.[63,64] Some studies suggest that this class of medication might be effective in patients with NAR and infectious rhinitis.[65] Older antihistamines are associated with an undesirable sedative effect in some patients, whereas newer antihistamines are less sedating.[66] Antihistamines can also be administered intranasally, with the advantage of a more rapid onset but with a shorter duration of action.[7] Antihistamines are currently permitted for use under the WADA's regulations.[59]

Cromoglycate is a mast cell stabilizer that can be used intranasally to reduce rhinorrhea, sneezing, and/or itching. Cromolyns are safe but have short half-lives and must be taken for several days to control exercise-related symptoms. The role of mast cells in relation to local epithelial dysfunction and exercise-induced airway disease has previously been demonstrated.[67,68] Cromolyns are currently permitted for use under the WADA's regulations.[59]

Antileukotrienes

Leukotriene receptor antagonists (LTRAs) have been shown to reduce nasal symptoms in patients with allergic rhinitis. LTRAs are a nonsedating alternative to common antihistamines.[63] LTRAs do not have any particular side effects in relation to exercise.[69] LTRAs are currently permitted for use under the WADA's regulations.[59]

Intranasal Corticosteroids

Nasal corticosteroids are also a first-line treatment option for allergic rhinitis because of their strong antiinflammatory effect. Nasal corticosteroids have been proven effective and are superior to oral antihistamines in reducing nasal obstruction.[70,71] In athletes with NAR or chronic rhinosinusitis, intranasal corticosteroids are the therapy of choice. The most common side effects of intranasal corticosteroids are epistaxis, irritation of the throat and nose, and nasal dryness.[72] Although oral, intravenous, intramuscular, or rectal corticosteroids are prohibited in competition only by the WADA's regulations, nasal corticosteroids are currently permitted.[59]

Decongestants

Decongestants relieve sino-nasal congestion and are effective in treating symptoms related to infectious as well as mild intermittent allergic rhinitis, if used on a short-term basis.[7] Common problems associated with decongestants are a mild stimulant effect, tremor, insomnia, and a feeling of increased alertness. Decongestants can also elevate heart rate and blood pressure, a potential problem for athletes with hypertensive issues. Long-term usage of decongestant nasal sprays can result in a rebound effect, leading to an increase in nasal mucosa congestion when the decongestive effect wears off.[73] Hence, in the absence of any contraindication, the use of decongestants should be limited to about 1 week. The use of many decongestants containing sympathomimetic amines or stimulants is currently prohibited or prohibited in competition only according to the WADA's regulations, and current knowledge of regulations is strongly recommended when prescribing such medications.[59]

Immunotherapy

Allergen immunotherapy represents a valuable option in athletes with allergic rhinitis, given the potential long-term induction of immune tolerance with regression of symptoms,[74] the current safety profiles of sublingual and subcutaneous formulations, and the fact that immunotherapy is currently permitted by the WADA's regulations.[59] It is recommended to start immunotherapy outside the competitive season because it can be accompanied by local or even systemic side effects, mostly during the start-up phase of the treatment.[75] Strenuous exercise should be avoided in the hours after the injection or intake, as this increases the risk for systemic side effects.[74]

SUMMARY

Proper sino-nasal function is important for athletes. Sino-nasal disease has been frequently reported in elite athletes and negatively impacts quality of life and sport performance. The mechanisms leading to exercise-induced sino-nasal disease in athletes are still poorly understood. In view of the united airway disease concept, sino-nasal disease is considered to be a risk factor for the persistence of lower airway symptoms and asthma; therefore, early diagnosis and treatment of sino-nasal symptoms are crucial for athletes in order to control their respiratory function and minimalize the effect on their athletic performance.

ACKNOWLEDGMENTS

The authors would like to thank Professor Emeritus Jan Ceuppens (KU Leuven, Belgium) for his scientific advice and carefully reviewing the document.

REFERENCES

1. World_Health_Organization. Global recommendations on physical activity for health. 2010; Available at: http://apps.who.int/iris/bitstream/10665/44399/1/9789241599979_eng.pdf. Accessed July 10, 2017.
2. Doulaptsi M, Steelant B, Hellings PW. Treating the nose for controlling the lung: a vanishing story?. In: Bachert C, Bourdin A, Chanez P, editors. The Nose and Sinuses in Respiratory Disorders (ERS Monograph). Sheffield (UK): European Respiratory Society; 2017.
3. Walker A, Surda P, Rossiter M, et al. Nasal function and dysfunction in exercise. J Laryngol Otol 2016;130(5):431–4.
4. Katz RM. Rhinitis in the athlete. J Allergy Clin Immunol 1984;73(5 Pt 2):708–11.
5. Ondolo C, Aversa S, Passali F, et al. Nasal and lung function in competitive swimmers. Acta Otorhinolaryngol Ital 2009;29(3):137–43.
6. Hox V, Maes T, Huvenne W, et al. A chest physician's guide to mechanisms of sinonasal disease. Thorax 2015;70(4):353–8.
7. Bousquet J, Khaltaev N, Cruz AA, et al. Allergic Rhinitis and its Impact on Asthma (ARIA) 2008 update (in collaboration with the World Health Organization, GA(2) LEN and AllerGen). Allergy 2008;63(Suppl 86):8–160.
8. Meltzer EO. Quality of life in adults and children with allergic rhinitis. J Allergy Clin Immunol 2001;108(1 Suppl):S45–53.
9. Fokkens WJ, Lund VJ, Mullol J, et al. EPOS 2012: European position paper on rhinosinusitis and nasal polyps 2012. A summary for otorhinolaryngologists. Rhinology 2012;50(1):1–12.
10. Hastan D, Fokkens WJ, Bachert C, et al. Chronic rhinosinusitis in Europe–an underestimated disease. A GA(2)LEN study. Allergy 2011;66(9):1216–23.
11. Bonini M, Gramiccioni C, Fioretti D, et al. Asthma, allergy and the Olympics: a 12-year survey in elite athletes. Curr Opin Allergy Clin Immunol 2015;15(2):184–92.
12. Fregosi RF, Lansing RW. Neural drive to nasal dilator muscles: influence of exercise intensity and oronasal flow partitioning. J Appl Physiol (1985) 1995;79(4):1330–7.
13. Kippelen P, Fitch KD, Anderson SD, et al. Respiratory health of elite athletes - preventing airway injury: a critical review. Br J Sports Med 2012;46(7):471–6.
14. Seys SF, Hox V, Van Gerven L, et al. Damage-associated molecular pattern and innate cytokine release in the airways of competitive swimmers. Allergy 2015;70(2):187–94.
15. Hallstrand TS, Moody MW, Wurfel MM, et al. Inflammatory basis of exercise-induced bronchoconstriction. Am J Respir Crit Care Med 2005;172(6):679–86.
16. Bonini S, Bonini M, Bousquet J, et al. Rhinitis and asthma in athletes: an ARIA document in collaboration with GA2LEN. Allergy 2006;61(6):681–92.

17. Spence L, Brown WJ, Pyne DB, et al. Incidence, etiology, and symptomatology of upper respiratory illness in elite athletes. Med Sci Sports Exerc 2007;39(4): 577–86.
18. Schwartz LB, Delgado L, Craig T, et al. Exercise-induced hypersensitivity syndromes in recreational and competitive athletes: a PRACTALL consensus report (what the general practitioner should know about sports and allergy). Allergy 2008;63(8):953–61.
19. Thomas S, Wolfarth B, Wittmer C, et al, study-Team GA-O. Self-reported asthma and allergies in top athletes compared to the general population - results of the German part of the GA2LEN-Olympic study 2008. Allergy Asthma Clin Immunol 2010;6(1):31.
20. Katelaris CH, Carrozzi FM, Burke TV, et al. Patterns of allergic reactivity and disease in Olympic athletes. Clin J Sport Med 2006;16(5):401–5.
21. Alaranta A, Alaranta H, Heliovaara M, et al. Allergic rhinitis and pharmacological management in elite athletes. Med Sci Sports Exerc 2005;37(5):707–11.
22. Weiler JM, Layton T, Hunt M. Asthma in United States Olympic athletes who participated in the 1996 Summer Games. J Allergy Clin Immunol 1998;102(5): 722–6.
23. Nieman DC. Exercise, upper respiratory tract infection, and the immune system. Med Sci Sports Exerc 1994;26(2):128–39.
24. Reeser JC, Willick S, Elstad M. Medical services provided at the Olympic Village polyclinic during the 2002 Salt Lake City Winter Games. WMJ 2003;102(4):20–5.
25. Robinson D, Milne C. Medicine at the 2000 Sydney Olympic Games: the New Zealand health team. Br J Sports Med 2002;36(3):229.
26. Nieman DC, Johanssen LM, Lee JW, et al. Infectious episodes in runners before and after the Los Angeles Marathon. J Sports Med Phys Fitness 1990,30(3): 316–28.
27. Peters EM, Bateman ED. Ultramarathon running and upper respiratory tract infections. An epidemiological survey. S Afr Med J 1983;64(15):582–4.
28. Cox AJ, Gleeson M, Pyne DB, et al. Clinical and laboratory evaluation of upper respiratory symptoms in elite athletes. Clin J Sport Med 2008;18(5):438–45.
29. Brozek JL, Bousquet J, Baena-Cagnani CE, et al. Allergic Rhinitis and its Impact on Asthma (ARIA) guidelines: 2010 revision. J Allergy Clin Immunol 2010;126(3): 466–76.
30. Helenius IJ, Tikkanen HO, Sarna S, et al. Asthma and increased bronchial responsiveness in elite athletes: atopy and sport event as risk factors. J Allergy Clin Immunol 1998;101(5):646–52.
31. Katelaris CH, Carrozzi FM, Burke TV, et al. A springtime Olympics demands special consideration for allergic athletes. J Allergy Clin Immunol 2000;106(2):260–6.
32. Lappuci G, Rasi G, Bonini S, et al. Allergy and infectious diseases in athletes. J Allergy Clin Immunol 2003;11(2 Suppl 1):S142.
33. Hellings PW, Klimek L, Cingi C, et al. Non-allergic rhinitis: position paper of the European Academy of Allergy and Clinical Immunology. Allergy 2017;72(11): 1657–65.
34. Walker A, Surda P, Rossiter M, et al. Rhinitis in elite and non-elite field hockey players. Int J Sports Med 2017;38(1):65–70.
35. Van Gerven L, Boeckxstaens G, Jorissen M, et al. Short-time cold dry air exposure: a useful diagnostic tool for nasal hyperresponsiveness. Laryngoscope 2012;122(12):2615–20.
36. Gerth van Wijk RG, de Graaf-in 't Veld C, Garrelds IM. Nasal hyperreactivity. Rhinology 1999;37(2):50–5.

37. Bonadonna P, Senna G, Zanon P, et al. Cold-induced rhinitis in skiers–clinical aspects and treatment with ipratropium bromide nasal spray: a randomized controlled trial. Am J Rhinol 2001;15(5):297–301.
38. Passali D, Damiani V, Passali GC, et al. Alterations in rhinosinusal homeostasis in a sportive population: our experience with 106 athletes. Eur Arch Otorhinolaryngol 2004;261(9):502–6.
39. Langdeau JB, Turcotte H, Bowie DM, et al. Airway hyperresponsiveness in elite athletes. Am J Respir Crit Care Med 2000;161(5):1479–84.
40. Gelardi M, Ventura MT, Fiorella R, et al. Allergic and non-allergic rhinitis in swimmers: clinical and cytological aspects. Br J Sports Med 2012;46(1):54–8.
41. Levesque B, Duchesne JF, Gingras S, et al. The determinants of prevalence of health complaints among young competitive swimmers. Int Arch Occup Environ Health 2006;80(1):32–9.
42. Zwick H, Popp W, Budik G, et al. Increased sensitization to aeroallergens in competitive swimmers. Lung 1990;168(2):111–5.
43. Kohlhammer Y, Doring A, Schafer T, et al. Swimming pool attendance and hay fever rates later in life. Allergy 2006;61(11):1305–9.
44. Sonmez G, Uzun G, Mutluoglu M, et al. Paranasal sinus mucosal hypertrophy in experienced divers. Aviat Space Environ Med 2011;82(10):992–4.
45. Bougault V, Turmel J, St-Laurent J, et al. Asthma, airway inflammation and epithelial damage in swimmers and cold-air athletes. Eur Respir J 2009;33(4):740–6.
46. Muns G, Rubinstein I, Singer P. Neutrophil chemotactic activity is increased in nasal secretions of long-distance runners. Int J Sports Med 1996;17(1):56–9.
47. Muns G, Singer P, Wolf F, et al. Impaired nasal mucociliary clearance in long-distance runners. Int J Sports Med 1995;16(4):209–13.
48. Cavalcante de Sa M, Nakagawa NK, Saldiva de Andre CD, et al. Aerobic exercise in polluted urban environments: effects on airway defense mechanisms in young healthy amateur runners. J Breath Res 2016;10(4):046018.
49. Lakier Smith L. Overtraining, excessive exercise, and altered immunity: is this a T helper-1 versus T helper-2 lymphocyte response? Sports Med 2003;33(5):347–64.
50. Steensberg A, Toft AD, Bruunsgaard H, et al. Strenuous exercise decreases the percentage of type 1 T cells in the circulation. J Appl Physiol (1985) 2001;91(4):1708–12.
51. Dallimore NS, Eccles R. Changes in human nasal resistance associated with exercise, hyperventilation and rebreathing. Acta Otolaryngol 1977;84(5–6):416–21.
52. Anderson SD, Daviskas E. The mechanism of exercise-induced asthma is. J Allergy Clin Immunol 2000;106(3):453–9.
53. Bernard A. Chlorination products: emerging links with allergic diseases. Curr Med Chem 2007;14(16):1771–82.
54. Stanford CF, Stanford RL. Exercise induced rhinorrhoea (athlete's nose). BMJ 1988;297(6649):660.
55. Hellings PW, Scadding G, Alobid I, et al. Executive summary of European Task Force document on diagnostic tools in rhinology. Rhinology 2012;50(4):339–52.
56. Couto M, Kurowski M, Moreira A, et al. Mechanisms of exercise-induced bronchoconstriction in athletes: current perspectives and future challenges. Allergy 2018;73(1):8–16.
57. Pyne DB, McDonald WA, Gleeson M, et al. Mucosal immunity, respiratory illness, and competitive performance in elite swimmers. Med Sci Sports Exerc 2001;33(3):348–53.

58. Pyne DB, Hopkins WG, Batterham AM, et al. Characterising the individual performance responses to mild illness in international swimmers. Br J Sports Med 2005; 39(10):752–6.
59. World_Anti-Doping_Agency. The world anti-doping code international standard. Prohibited list: January, 2017. 2017: Available at: https://www.wada-ama.org/sites/default/files/resources/files/2016-09-29_-_wada_prohibited_list_2017_eng_final.pdf. Accessed June 27, 2017.
60. Organization WH. Guidelines for safe recreational water environments. Volume 2: swimming pools and similar environments. 2006. p. xviii. Available at: http://www.who.int/water_sanitation_health/bathing/srwe2full.pdf. Accessed June 27, 2017.
61. Fantuzzi G, Righi E, Predieri G, et al. Airborne trichloramine (NCl(3)) levels and self-reported health symptoms in indoor swimming pool workers: dose-response relationships. J Expo Sci Environ Epidemiol 2013;23(1):88–93.
62. Seys SF, Feyen L, Keirsbilck S, et al. An outbreak of swimming-pool related respiratory symptoms: an elusive source of trichloramine in a municipal indoor swimming pool. Int J Hyg Environ Health 2015;218(4):386–91.
63. Wei C. The efficacy and safety of H1-antihistamine versus montelukast for allergic rhinitis: a systematic review and meta-analysis. Biomed Pharmacother 2016;83: 989–97.
64. Xu Y, Zhang J, Wang J. The efficacy and safety of selective H1-antihistamine versus leukotriene receptor antagonist for seasonal allergic rhinitis: a meta-analysis. PLoS One 2014;9(11):e112815.
65. De Sutter AI, Saraswat A, van Driel ML. Antihistamines for the common cold. Cochrane Database Syst Rev 2015;(11):CD009345.
66. Passalacqua G, Bousquet J, Bachert C, et al. The clinical safety of H1-receptor antagonists. An EAACI position paper. Allergy 1996;51(10):666–75.
67. Kippelen P, Larsson J, Anderson SD, et al. Effect of sodium cromoglycate on mast cell mediators during hyperpnea in athletes. Med Sci Sports Exerc 2010; 42(10):1853–60.
68. Hallstrand TS, Altemeier WA, Aitken ML, et al. Role of cells and mediators in exercise-induced bronchoconstriction. Immunol Allergy Clin North Am 2013; 33(3):313–28, vii.
69. Steinshamn S, Sandsund M, Sue-Chu M, et al. Effects of montelukast on physical performance and exercise economy in adult asthmatics with exercise-induced bronchoconstriction. Scand J Med Sci Sports 2002;12(4):211–7.
70. Juel-Berg N, Darling P, Bolvig J, et al. Intranasal corticosteroids compared with oral antihistamines in allergic rhinitis: a systematic review and meta-analysis. Am J Rhinol Allergy 2017;31(1):19–28.
71. Okano M. Mechanisms and clinical implications of glucocorticosteroids in the treatment of allergic rhinitis. Clin Exp Immunol 2009;158(2):164–73.
72. Sastre J, Mosges R. Local and systemic safety of intranasal corticosteroids. J Investig Allergol Clin Immunol 2012;22(1):1–12.
73. Greiner AN, Hellings PW, Rotiroti G, et al. Allergic rhinitis. Lancet 2011;378(9809): 2112–22.
74. Keles N. Treating allergic rhinitis in the athlete. Rhinology 2002;40(4):211–4.
75. Katelaris CH, Carrozzi FM, Burke TV. Allergic rhinoconjunctivitis in elite athletes: optimal management for quality of life and performance. Sports Med 2003;33(6): 401–6.
76. Fayock K, Voltz M, Sandella B, et al. Antibiotic precautions in athletes. Sports Health 2014;6(4):321–5.

Exercise-Induced Laryngeal Obstruction—An Overview

Leif Nordang, MD, PhD[a], Katarina Norlander, MD, PhD[a],
Emil Schwarz Walsted, MD, PhD[b,c],*

KEYWORDS

- Exercise • Larynx • Airway obstruction • Exercise-induced laryngeal obstruction
- Continuous laryngoscopy during exercise

KEY POINTS

- Exercise-induced laryngeal obstruction (EILO) is a prevalent cause of exertional dyspnea and is frequently noted in adolescent girls.
- Advances in EILO diagnostics have led to the distinction of EILO from other forms of inducible laryngeal obstruction.
- Although multiple anatomic phenotypes of EILO have been visually identified, understanding of EILO pathophysiology and mechanism remains limited.

BACKGROUND AND HISTORICAL OVERVIEW

Exercise-induced laryngeal obstruction (EILO) describes conditions in which the laryngeal inlet closes partially or completely during exercise. Patients with EILO clinically present with exertional dyspnea with or without stridor. Although frequently mistaken for, or coexistent with, exercise-induced asthma, it is a distinct entity,[1,2] and its importance and improved recognition have only really become apparent over the past few decades.

Inducible laryngeal obstruction (ILO) unrelated to exercise was first described in the nineteenth century. For more than 100 years, in part due to a lack of diagnostic modalities that could easily characterize anatomy during periods of respiratory distress, publications devoted to the condition focused on case reports and speculative theories about disease mechanism. Initially described as "hysterical croup in women" and "Munchausen stridor," psychological mechanisms were widely accepted as the cause of stridor and dyspnea.[3–6]

The authors have no real or perceived conflicts of interest.
[a] Department of Surgical Sciences, Otorhinolaryngology and Head and Neck Surgery, Uppsala University, Sjukhusvägen 85, 751 85 Uppsala, Sweden; [b] Respiratory Research Unit, Department of Respiratory Medicine, Bispebjerg University Hospital, Bispebjerg Bakke 23, Copenhagen DK-2400, Denmark; [c] Respiratory Department, Royal Brompton Hospital, Dovehouse Street, SW3 6JY, London, UK
* Corresponding author.
E-mail address: emilwalsted@dadlnet.dk

Immunol Allergy Clin N Am 38 (2018) 271–280
https://doi.org/10.1016/j.iac.2018.01.001
0889-8561/18/© 2018 Elsevier Inc. All rights reserved.

immunology.theclinics.com

The development of fiber-optic endoscopic technology in the 1960s facilitated examination of the larynx in patients suffering from laryngeal symptoms. In 1982, Chung[7] reported that laryngeal symptoms could mimic the presentation of acute asthma. This was followed by descriptions from Christopher and colleagues,[8] who coined the term, *vocal cord dysfunction (VCD)*, and Lakin and colleagues,[9] who detailed inappropriate laryngeal closure occurring in relation to exercise based on a fiber-optic laryngeal evaluation after exercise. This early work, which relied on visual findings, highlighted the anatomic contribution to disease and led to the recognition of ILO as an entity distinct from asthma.

More than a decade later, in the mid-1990s, Smith and colleagues,[10] followed by Bent and colleagues,[11] Beaty and colleagues,[12] and Naito and Niimi,[13] visualized the larynx during exercise. By studying the larynx during exercise, new insights into subtypes of EILO were attained. In addition to other case reports and series describing inappropriate glottic adduction during exercise, visual data obtained during exercise led to the realization that the supraglottic structures could partially or fully obstruct the laryngeal inlet with little or no involvement of the vocal folds. This specific phenomenon was termed, *exercise-induced laryngomalacia*, due to the anatomic resemblance with congenital laryngomalacia.[10]

In 2006, Heimdal and colleagues[14] presented a formal description of a novel clinical methodology, describing continuous laryngoscopy during a standardized treadmill exercise test. This test, termed, *continuous laryngoscopy exercise (CLE) test*, provided researchers and clinicians with a procedural framework for EILO diagnosis and enabled laryngeal video recording during exercise. The CLE test has been subsequently adapted to different exercise modalities[15–17] and is now considered the gold standard for the diagnosis of EILO.[18] This is important because descriptions and future studies of EILO epidemiology, conditions associated with the disease, mechanism, and response to various therapies depend on robust objective diagnostic methodologies.

The CLE test has facilitated improved understanding of different anatomic phenotypes of EILO (**Fig. 1**A). Recent work has demonstrated that laryngeal obstruction can occur at the glottic level (ie, the vocal folds adduct [**Fig. 1**C]) or at the supraglottic level (ie, closure caused by prolapse of the arytenoid cartilages aryepiglottic fold [**Fig. 1**B]). At times, the obstruction is caused by a combination of glottic and supraglottic obstruction (**Fig. 1**D) and in rare cases, a retroflexion of the epiglottis may occlude the laryngeal inlet (**Fig. 1**E).[19]

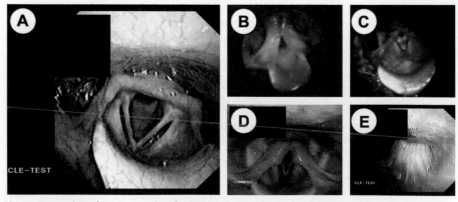

Fig. 1. Examples of EILO. Panel A depicts Normal. All images depict the larynx in inspiration during exercise. (*B*) Supraglottic. (*C*) Glottic. (*D*) Combined glottis and supraglottic. (*E*) Retroflexing epiglottis.

In the past few decades, multiple therapeutic options have evolved, guided mainly by theory and clinical experience. These are detailed in subsequent articles of this edition. Management options include respiratory retraining and voice therapy as guided by speech-language pathologists,[8,20,21] breathing pattern modification,[8,22,23] inspiratory muscle training,[24-26] psychological intervention, and surgery.[27-30]

NOMENCLATURE

Over the past several decades, EILO has been labeled by many terms. The lack of international consensus terminology in this area has undoubtedly confounded both clinical and research progress in the field. Early labels, including "hysterical croup," "Munchausen stridor," and "factitious asthma," may have stigmatized the condition and implied a purely psychological or factitious mechanism to the condition. Other terms, such as VCD and paradoxic vocal fold motion, provided a less judgmental label but did not distinguish patients with isolated exercise symptoms from others. Later, the prefix "exercise-induced" was used to draw attention to a subset of patients affected during exercise only. Along with these terms, dozens of other terms have appeared in the literature over the past few decades, causing a degree of confusion as to whether EILO is 1 entity or many and whether EILO is distinct from episodic upper airway obstruction caused by other triggers.

To address terminology confusion in the literature and provide guidance for clinicians and researchers, a joint American College of Chest Physicians, European Respiratory Society, and European Laryngological Society task force was formed to establish a consensus report on nomenclature.[18] This report introduced the broad umbrella term, ILO, to denominate laryngeal closure induced by a trigger. Exercise was identified as 1 of many triggers, with EILO identified as a distinct entity. This same task force also advocated for the use of descriptors of the time course and anatomic location of visualized obstruction to be included to facilitate future comparisons of studies. The entire nomenclature, as proposed by the task force, has not yet been widely adopted and, as a recent communication mentions, this may be due to the complexity of recording such a description.[31]

EPIDEMIOLOGY

The 2 population-based studies relying on endoscopic diagnosis published to date[2,32] identify the prevalence of EILO as 5% to 7% among adolescents and young adults, a figure much nearer asthma prevalence than previously appreciated. There are no definitive data that characterize population prevalence in samples balanced across the age spectrum. With respect to the effect of gender on EILO prevalence, case series data suggest that EILO is more common in the female gender than in the male[18] (**Table 1**). In population-based studies, Christensen and colleagues[32] also reported a higher prevalence among girls and women whereas Johansson and colleagues[2] did not in population-based studies. Precise data on the effect of race and ethnicity on EILO prevalence are also not published, although some series report a very high proportion of caucasian patients.[33,34]

NORMAL UPPER AIRWAY FUNCTION AND PROPOSED EXERCISE-INDUCED LARYNGEAL OBSTRUCTION PATHOPHYSIOLOGY

It is essential to understand normal upper airway function to study disease mechanism in EILO. The larynx serves several different purposes: it takes part in breathing, produces voice, protects the airway from aspiration, assists in swallowing, and

Table 1
Recent studies describing basic epidemiologic data on exercise-induced laryngeal obstruction

Author(s)	N	Study Description	Proportion with Moderate or Severe Exercise-Induced Laryngeal Obstruction	Gender Distribution of Subjects with Exercise-Induced Laryngeal Obstruction	Age
Roksund et al,[19] 2009	171	Case-control study examining selected patients with exertional dyspnea in a tertiary clinic	66% of tested 78% of analyzable tests	72% female	Mean ± SD 16.3 ± 7.3
Christensen et al,[32] 2011	98	Cross-sectional examining young and adolescent general population	43% of tested 7.6% of invited	Female: male OR 3.41	Median (range) 19 (14–24)
Nielsen et al,[1] 2013	88	Retrospective chart review of athletes referred to CLE in a tertiary asthma clinic	35%	77% female	Median (IQR) 18 (11)
Tilles et al,[52] 2013	143	Retrospective chart review of patients with EILO confirmed by postexercise laryngoscopy	100% (by design)	77% female	Mean ± SD 14 ± 2.6
Johansson et al,[2] 2015	125	Cross-sectional investigation of young general population participants with exertional dyspnea	7% of tested 5.4% of population	66% female	Mean (range) 14.2 (13–15)
Hilland et al,[53] 2016	20	Case-control study of patients admitted to hospital for congenital laryngomalacia	70% of cases 10% of controls	66% female	Mean ± SD 12.7 ± 2.7
Olin et al,[33] 2016	71	Adolescents and young adults referred to a specialist center for CLE on suspicion of EILO	75%	66% female	Mean ± SD 15 ± 2
Olin et al,[34] 2016	36	Subjects with EILO refractory to conventional respiratory retraining and other therapies	100% (by design)	78% female	Mean ± SD 17 ± 3.5
Buchvald et al,[54] 2016	54	Consecutively CLE-tested children at a tertiary center	35%	61% female	Mean ± SD 13.4 ± 2.0
Hseu et al,[55] 2016	290	Retrospective chart review of patients with suspected EILO (PVFMD) at a tertiary clinic	30%	77% female	Mean ± SD 15.4 ± 2.5

Study	N	Population		% female	Age
Walsted et al,[56] 2017	37	Patients with suspected asthma and exertional dyspnea consecutively referred to a tertiary asthma clinic	22%	100% female	Median (IQR) 22.5 (12)
Hočevar-Boltežar et al,[57] 2017	59	Adolescents and young adults referred for laryngeal hypersensitivity testing at a specialist center	100% (by design)	69% female	Mean ± SD 24.3 ± 2.8
Walsted et al,[58] 2017	38	Subjects with EILO and healthy controls willing to undergo 4 consecutive CLE tests	74% (by design)	83% female	Mean ± SD 23 (15–45)
Walsted et al,[59] 2017	38	Ten patients with EILO and their family members willing to undergo CLE testing	37% of tested 25% of family members	86% female	N/A

Abbreviations: IQR, interquartile range; PVFMD, paradoxic vocal fold movement disorder.

participates in clearing the airway via cough. During exercise, a key role of the larynx is to maintain airway patency and facilitate increased ventilation. In healthy individuals, this is accomplished through vocal fold abduction, which maximizes the size of the laryngeal inlet and the rima glottidis. Additionally, with increased airflow, the epiglottis is tilted anteriorly toward the base of the tongue, further increasing the cross-sectional area of the laryngeal inlet (**Fig. 2**). Although several muscles take part in adducting the vocal folds and thereby decrease the rima glottidis, abduction of the vocal folds is the result of contraction of only 1 muscle, the posterior cricoarytenoid (PCA) muscle.[35]

In cases of EILO, dynamic obstruction can be observed at the glottic or supraglottic level (rarely including the epiglottis).[19] Supraglottic obstruction seems to most often precede inspiratory glottic narrowing during incremental exercise challenges and seems to occur almost exclusively during inspiration.[19] Glottic obstruction is most prominent during inspiration, although expiratory obstruction may be present and is recognized to occur in chronic obstructive pulmonary diseas.[36]

The impact of observed laryngeal obstruction on symptom generation may vary across patients. In severe cases, this obstruction can be associated with impaired airflow, as measured by spirometry during exercise.[8,12,37] Several cases of EILO have been described, however, in association with apparently normal airflow during exercise.[38,39] In patients with apparently normal airflow (as well as in patients with inspiratory airflow limitation), it is hypothesized that respiratory muscle work increases greatly in EILO to optimize inspiratory airflow. In addition to changes in airflow, symptoms are an important domain of disease impact. There may be inhibitory or nociceptive effects from laryngeal closure, occurring independent of a significant reduction in measurable airflow related to alterations in airflow turbulence and sensory feedback. Additionally, some investigators have hypothesized that the sensations of dyspnea lead to panic-type reactions.[40]

Understanding of the mechanisms of EILO remains rudimentary. Differences in disease prevalence across epidemiologic strata may provide insight regarding disease mechanism. Additionally, different visualized anatomic phenotypes of EILO suggest that more than 1 pathophysiologic mechanism may exist. Finally, observations about associated conditions and behavioral traits of patients may shed light on disease mechanism. Several hypotheses regarding disease mechanism have been suggested.[18]

Laryngeal size may contribute to the presence or absence of disease. Patients with smaller airway dimensions may be more likely to experience EILO symptoms. Hormonal

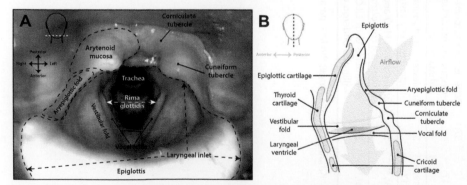

Fig. 2. Relevant anatomic structures and landmarks in the larynx in (*A*) axial plane (laryngoscopic view) and (*B*) midsagittal plane. Note the position of the cuneiform/corniculate tubercles and the aryepiglottic fold in relation to the vocal folds. (*From* Walsted ES. Evaluating diagnostic approaches in exercise-induced laryngeal obstruction. [Doctoral thesis]. Denmark: University of Copenhagen; 2017; with permission.)

changes during puberty mediate differential laryngeal growth across gender. The laryngeal diameter of adult women is smaller than that of adult men.[41,42] Such an explanation could explain the high proportion of adolescent girls in EILO samples.

The structural integrity of supraglottic tissues may contribute to disease. Based on visual observations, it is hypothesized that supraglottic EILO is a partially passive phenomenon in which increasing exertion and ventilation increases the negative transmural pressure.[40] When the inward-pulling forces caused by this negative pressure become greater than the outward-pulling forces of the supporting tissue (ie, muscles and connective tissue), an inward collapse occurs.[19,29] This movement is likely accentuated by the Venturi effect (ie, a further increase in negative pressure as a result of a choked section of the airway and consequently higher air velocity at the site of obstruction). In healthy individuals, rigid cartilage, strong connective tissue, and active laryngeal and pharyngeal muscles counteract the increasingly negative pressure created by maximal ventilation. It is conceivable that inflammatory processes or neuromuscular defects could alter the mechanical properties of these structures. Decreased strength of muscles or increased laxity of connective tissue might also explain why the upper airway lumen decreases with age in adults.[42]

Increased tone of specific structures may contribute to disease in certain individuals. In exercise, the epiglottis moves anteriorly, potentially increasing tension in the aryepiglottic folds.[43] This phenomenon may augment supraglottic closure in cases characterized by high baseline the aryepiglottic fold tension as these structures may consequently pull the arytenoid mucosa anteriorly, decreasing the size of the laryngeal inlet (see **Fig. 2**).

An imbalance of laryngeal abductors and adductors may also contribute to disease. Inappropriate glottic closure can be caused either by failure of the PCA itself to maintain abduction or by an imbalance in adductor and PCA activity or strength, leading to greater adduction than abduction forces (as seen in adductor spasmodic dysphonia).[44,45] Upper airway reactivity mediated by neuromuscular mechanisms may play a role. The glottic closure reflex serves to protect the lower airways against aspiration; thus, reflex sensitization as a consequence of laryngeal hypersensitivity could explain this inappropriate adduction.[46–48]

Behavioral health considerations have been associated with EILO, although causal relationships with respect to disease mechanism are unclear.[49] Anxiety-spectrum pathology and perfectionistic tendencies have been described in EILO patients.[50,51] It is possible that some of the signaling mechanisms that predispose to these behavioral findings contribute to disease mechanism. It is also possible that symptoms lead to specific behavioral changes.

Independent of anatomic, physiologic, and behavioral considerations, lifestyle choices may affect disease prevalence. In adolescence, some individuals become more active in sports and thus experience an increased demand for ventilation. This might explain why EILO usually debuts in adolescence or young adulthood. Additionally, there is some evidence that respiratory symptoms and visualized EILO grade score decrease with increasing age.[29] Some investigators hypothesize that this attenuation is due to a change in exercise habits,[29,30] with an understanding that older individuals are less likely to experience EILO because it is an effort-dependent condition.[33]

SUMMARY

In summary, EILO is a prevalent condition causing exertional breathlessness. It is distinct from asthma, often mistaken for asthma, and may coexist with asthma. Since its recognition, as a clinical entity in the 1980s, understanding of anatomic disease features has improved. CLE is now considered the gold standard for diagnosing EILO. The use of this procedure has led to differentiation of common subtypes of the condition: a glottic type (closure of the vocal folds themselves), a supraglottic type (arytenoid and aryepiglottic mucosa obstructing the laryngeal inlet), and a combination of the 2. Current understanding of disease mechanisms is basic, although anatomic observations as well as observations of the high proportion of adolescent female patients may guide initial studies.

REFERENCES

1. Nielsen EW, Hull JH, Backer V. High prevalence of exercise-induced laryngeal obstruction in athletes. Med Sci Sports Exerc 2013;45(11):2030–5.
2. Johansson H, Norlander K, Berglund L, et al. Prevalence of exercise-induced bronchoconstriction and exercise-induced laryngeal obstruction in a general adolescent population. Thorax 2015;70(1):57–63.
3. Dunglison R. The practice of medicine, vol. 2. Philadelphia: Lea & Blanchard; 1842. p. 321–2.
4. Hull JH, Selby J, Sandhu G. "You say potato, I say potato": time for consensus in exercise-induced laryngeal obstruction? Otolaryngol Head Neck Surg 2014; 151(5):891–2.
5. Patterson R, Schatz M, Horton M. Munchausen's stridor: non-organic laryngeal obstruction. Clin Allergy 1974;4(3):307–10.
6. Downing ET, Braman SS, Fox MJ, et al. Factitious asthma: physiological approach to diagnosis. JAMA 1982;248(21):2878–81.
7. Chung KF. Laryngeal stridor during acute asthma. Lancet 1982;2(8301):767.
8. Christopher KL, Wood RP, Eckert RC, et al. Vocal-cord dysfunction presenting as asthma. N Engl J Med 1983;308(26):1566–70.
9. Lakin RC, Metzger WJ, Haughey BH. Upper airway obstruction presenting as exercise-induced asthma. Chest 1984;86(3):499–501.
10. Smith RJH, Kramer M, Bauman NM, et al. Exercise-induced laryngomalacia. Ann Otol Rhinol Laryngol 1995;104(7):537–41.
11. Bent JP, Miller DA, Kim JW, et al. Pediatric exercise-induced laryngomalacia. Ann Otol Rhinol Laryngol 1996;105(3):169–75.
12. Beaty MM, Wilson JS, Smith RJH. Laryngeal motion during exercise. Laryngoscope 1999;109(1):136–9.
13. Naito A, Niimi S. The larynx during exercise. Laryngoscope 2000;110(7):1147–50.
14. Heimdal J-H, Roksund OD, Halvorsen T, et al. Continuous laryngoscopy exercise test: a method for visualizing laryngeal dysfunction during exercise. Laryngoscope 2006;116(1):52–7.
15. Tervonen H, Niskanen MM, Sovijärvi AR, et al. Fiberoptic videolaryngoscopy during bicycle ergometry: a diagnostic tool for exercise-induced vocal cord dysfunction. Laryngoscope 2009;119(9):1776–80.
16. Panchasara B, Nelson C, Niven R, et al. Lesson of the month: rowing-induced laryngeal obstruction: a novel cause of exertional dyspnoea: characterised by direct laryngoscopy. Thorax 2015;70(1):95–7.
17. Walsted ES, Swanton LL, van van Someren K, et al. Laryngoscopy during swimming: a novel diagnostic technique to characterize swimming- induced laryngeal obstruction. Laryngoscope 2017. https://doi.org/10.1002/lary.26532.
18. Halvorsen T, Walsted ES, Bucca C, et al. Inducible laryngeal obstruction (ILO) - an official joint European Respiratory Society and European Laryngological Society statement. Eur Respir J 2017;50. https://doi.org/10.1183/13993003.02221-2016.

19. Roksund OD, Maat RC, Heimdal J-H, et al. Exercise induced dyspnea in the young. Larynx as the bottleneck of the airways. Respir Med 2009;103(12): 1911–8.
20. Gallivan GJ, Hoffman L, Gallivan KH. Episodic paroxysmal laryngospasm: voice and pulmonary function assessment and management. J Voice 1996;10(1):93–105.
21. Andrianopoulos MV, Gallivan GJ, Gallivan KH. PVCM, PVCD, EPL, and irritable larynx syndrome: what are we talking about and how do we treat it? J Voice 2000;14(4):607–18.
22. Newsham KR, Klaben BK, Miller VJ, et al. Paradoxical vocal-cord dysfunction: management in athletes. J Athl Train 2002;37(3):325–8.
23. Rameau A, Foltz RS, Wagner K, et al. Multidisciplinary approach to vocal cord dysfunction diagnosis and treatment in one session: a single institutional outcome study. Int J Pediatr Otorhinolaryngol 2012;76(1):31–5.
24. Archer GJ, Hoyle JL, McCluskey A, et al. Inspiratory vocal cord dysfunction, a new approach in treatment. Eur Respir J 2000;15(3):617.
25. Mathers-Schmidt BA, Brilla LR. Inspiratory muscle training in exercise-induced paradoxical vocal fold motion. J Voice 2005;19(4):635–44.
26. Sandnes A, Andersen T, Hilland M, et al. Laryngeal movements during inspiratory muscle training in healthy subjects. J Voice 2013;27(4):448–53.
27. Mehlum CS, Walsted ES, Godballe C, et al. Supraglottoplasty as treatment of exercise induced laryngeal obstruction (EILO). Eur Arch Otorhinolaryngol 2016; 273(4):945–51.
28. Maat RC, Roksund OD, Olofsson J, et al. Surgical treatment of exercise-induced laryngeal dysfunction. Eur Arch Otorhinolaryngol 2007;264(4):401–7.
29. Maat RC, Hilland M, Roksund OD, et al. Exercise-induced laryngeal obstruction: natural history and effect of surgical treatment. Eur Arch Otorhinolaryngol 2011; 268(10):1485–92.
30. Norlander K, Johansson H, Jansson C, et al. Surgical treatment is effective in severe cases of exercise-induced laryngeal obstruction: A follow-up study. Acta Otolaryngol 2015;135(11):1152–9.
31. Bardin PG, Low K, Ruane L, et al. Controversies and conundrums in vocal cord dysfunction. Lancet Respir Med 2017;5(7):546–8.
32. Christensen PM, Thomsen SF, Rasmussen N, et al. Exercise-induced laryngeal obstructions: prevalence and symptoms in the general public. Eur Arch Otorhinolaryngol 2011;268(9):1313–9.
33. Olin JT, Clary MS, Fan EM, et al. Continuous laryngoscopy quantitates laryngeal behaviour in exercise and recovery. Eur Respir J 2016;48(4):1192–200.
34. Olin JT, Deardorff EH, Fan EM, et al. Therapeutic laryngoscopy during exercise: a novel non-surgical therapy for refractory EILO. Pediatr Pulmonol 2016;24:445.
35. Zealear DL, Billante CR. Neurophysiology of vocal fold paralysis. Otolaryngol Clin North Am 2004;37(1):1–23.
36. Baz M, Haji GS, Menzies-Gow A, et al. Dynamic laryngeal narrowing during exercise: a mechanism for generating intrinsic PEEP in COPD? Thorax 2015;70(3):251–7.
37. Bittleman DB, Smith RJ, Weiler JM. Abnormal movement of the arytenoid region during exercise presenting as exercise-induced asthma in an adolescent athlete. Chest 1994;106(2):615–6.
38. Olin JT, Clary MS, Connors D, et al. Glottic configuration in patients with exercise-induced stridor: a new paradigm. Laryngoscope 2014;124(11):2568–73.
39. Christensen PM, Maltbæk N, Jørgensen IM, et al. Can flow-volume loops be used to diagnose exercise induced laryngeal obstructions? A comparison study

examining the accuracy and inter-rater agreement of flow volume loops as a diagnostic tool. Prim Care Respir J 2013;22(3):306–11.

40. Roksund OD, Heimdal J-H, Clemm H, et al. Exercise inducible laryngeal obstruction: diagnostics and management. Paediatr Respir Rev 2017;21:86–94.
41. Wysocki J, Kielska E, Orszulak P, et al. Measurements of pre- and postpubertal human larynx: a cadaver study. Surg Radiol Anat 2008;30(3):191–9.
42. Martin SE, Mathur R, Marshall I, et al. The effect of age, sex, obesity and posture on upper airway size. Eur Respir J 1997;10(9):2087–90.
43. Maat RC. Exercise-induced laryngeal obstruction - diagnostic procedures and therapy [Doctoral thesis]. University of Bergen, Norway; 2011.
44. Robe E, Brumlik J, Moore P. A study of spastic dysphonia. Neurologic and electroencephalographic abnormalities. Laryngoscope 1960;70:219–45.
45. Ludlow CL. Spasmodic dysphonia: a laryngeal control disorder specific to speech. J Neurosci 2011;31(3):793–7.
46. Aviv JE, Martin JH, Kim T, et al. Laryngopharyngeal sensory discrimination testing and the laryngeal adductor reflex. Ann Otol Rhinol Laryngol 1999;108(8):725–30.
47. Ludlow CL. Laryngeal reflexes: physiology, technique, and clinical use. J Clin Neurophysiol 2015;32(4):284–93.
48. Hull JH, Backer V, Gibson PG, et al. Laryngeal dysfunction - assessment and management for the clinician. Am J Respir Crit Care Med 2016;194(9):1062–72.
49. McFadden ER, Zawadski DK. Vocal cord dysfunction masquerading as exercise-induced asthma. a physiologic cause for "choking" during athletic activities. Am J Respir Crit Care Med 1996;153(3):942–7.
50. Husein OF, Husein TN, Gardner R, et al. Formal psychological testing in patients with paradoxical vocal fold dysfunction. Laryngoscope 2008;118(4):740–7.
51. Brugman SM, Simons SM. Vocal cord dysfunction: don't mistake it for asthma. Phys Sportsmed 1998;26(5):63–85.
52. Tilles SA, Ayars AG, Picciano JF, et al. Exercise-induced vocal cord dysfunction and exercise-induced laryngomalacia in children and adolescents: the same clinical syndrome? Ann Allergy Asthma Immunol 2013;111(5):342–6.e1.
53. Hilland M, Roksund OD, Sandvik L, et al. Congenital laryngomalacia is related to exercise-induced laryngeal obstruction in adolescence. Arch Dis Child 2016; 101(5):443–8.
54. Buchvald F, Phillipsen LD, Hjuler T, et al. Exercise-induced inspiratory symptoms in school children. Pediatr Pulmonol 2016;51(11):1200–5.
55. Hseu A, Sandler M, Ericson D, et al. Paradoxical vocal fold motion in children presenting with exercise induced dyspnea. Int J Pediatr Otorhinolaryngol 2016;90: 165–9.
56. Walsted ES, Hull JH, Sverrild A, et al. Bronchial provocation testing does not detect exercise-induced laryngeal obstruction. J Asthma 2017;54(1):77–83.
57. Hočevar-Boltežar I, Krivec U, Šereg-Bahar M. Laryngeal sensitivity testing in youth with exercise-inducible laryngeal obstruction. Int J Rehabil Res 2017;1. https://doi.org/10.1097/MRR.0000000000000222.
58. Walsted ES, Hull JH, Hvedstrup J, et al. Validity and reliability of grade scoring in the diagnosis of exercise-induced laryngeal obstruction. ERJ Open Res 2017; 3(3). https://doi.org/10.1183/23120541.00070-2017.
59. Walsted ES, Hvedstrup J, Eiberg H, et al. Heredity of supraglottic exercise-induced laryngeal obstruction. Eur Respir J 2017;50(2). https://doi.org/10.1183/13993003.00423-2017.

Working Towards a Common Transatlantic Approach for Evaluation of Exercise-Induced Laryngeal Obstruction

Ola Drange Røksund, DPT, PhD[a,b,*], J. Tod Olin, MD, MSCS[c],
Thomas Halvorsen, MD, PhD[b,d]

KEYWORDS

- Exercise-induced laryngeal obstruction (EILO)
- Continuous laryngoscopy during exercise (CLE)
- Exercise-induced bronchoconstriction (EIB)
- Exercise-induced inspiratory symptoms (EIIS) • Vocal cord dysfunction (VCD)

KEY POINTS

- The history is the key to a correct exercise-induced laryngeal obstruction (EILO) diagnosis, with inspiratory symptoms presenting during ongoing exercise and resolving within a few minutes after exercise termination.
- Exercise-induced inspiratory symptoms (EIIS) have multiple causes but are most often related to various forms of laryngeal obstruction; if so, the condition is labeled EILO.
- At present, no tools exist that can diagnose EILO at rest.
- Laryngoscopy performed as symptoms evolve, through the use of a procedure known as continuous laryngoscopy during exercise, is pivotal to patient workup.

Exertional dyspnea is a common presenting symptom among patients of general practitioners, respiratory specialists, allergists, otolaryngologists, cardiologists, and sports medicine specialists. The symptom complex is important as symptoms per se, as manifestations of systemic disease, and as a potential contributor to a sedentary lifestyle. Exertional dyspnea can be caused by a variety of conditions rooted in

Potential Conflict of Interest: Haukeland University Hospital owns part of US patent no. 11/134551, protecting the commercial rights of the CLE test.
Funding Information: Major Funding Institutions: Haukeland University Hospital, University of Bergen, and Bergen University College.
[a] The Faculty of Health and Social Sciences, Western Norway University of Applied Sciences, Bergen, Norway; [b] Department of Paediatrics, Haukeland University Hospital, Bergen, Norway; [c] Department of Pediatrics, National Jewish Health, Denver, Colorado, USA; [d] Department of Clinical Science, Section for Paediatrics, University of Bergen, Bergen, Norway
* Corresponding author. Høgskolen på Vestlandet, 7030, Bergen N-5020, Norway.
E-mail address: odro@hib.no

Immunol Allergy Clin N Am 38 (2018) 281–292
https://doi.org/10.1016/j.iac.2018.01.002
0889-8561/18/© 2018 The Authors. Published by Elsevier Inc. This is an open access article under the CC BY-NC-ND license (http://creativecommons.org/licenses/by-nc-nd/4.0/).

dysfunction of multiple organ systems and can be described variably by patients across etiologies.[1] Treatment depends on the cause of symptoms and may be simple, as in cases of mild exercise-induced asthma, or complex, as in cases of anemia caused by oncologic processes.

A malfunctioning larynx can be a source of exertional dyspnea. The larynx serves a variety of functions, and, in addition to moving in a precise manner to generate voice, it must accommodate between 100 L and 280 L per minute of airflow during intense exercise in adolescents and adults.[2] Exercise-induced laryngeal obstruction (EILO), the consensus term for the condition previously known as vocal cord dysfunction and paradoxic vocal fold motion, is defined by inappropriate narrowing of the larynx during high-intensity exercise.[3] First described in the 1980s as a mimic of asthma, EILO is an important condition for allergists and pulmonologists to consider because it is common in specific populations.[4] Recent studies from Scandinavian countries have highlighted the high prevalence of EILO in young and otherwise healthy young people, 5.7%[5] and 7.5%[6] of unselected adolescents in Uppsala, Sweden, and Copenhagen, Denmark, respectively. Studies of soldiers and athletes in stressful situations have revealed even higher rates.[7,8]

Given this high prevalence of EILO as well as its frequent misdiagnosis of asthma and the international effort stressing the importance of regular exercise for general health,[9] there is a need to develop diagnostic recommendations for the diagnosis of EILO.[10] A process to establish definitive diagnoses of EILO also serves other purposes. At an individual patient level, there is value in distinguishing EILO from asthma or other conditions to minimize unnecessary therapies, something commonly noted by investigators and also by the general press.[10-12] There is also value in distinguishing EILO patients from patients with other forms of inducible laryngeal obstruction (ILO) because there is important literature devoted to psychopathology in patients with resting symptoms, sometimes stigmatizing the diagnosis.[13-15] At the level of the medical provider community, streamlined recommendations are important because there is variability in terms of awareness of EILO across provider populations. As highlighted during discussions at the first international EILO conference in Bergen, Norway, April 2017, there is a perceived under-awareness of EILO within certain provider communities, but there is also a perception of EILO overdiagnosis which has led to EILO fatigue in other provider communities.

The recommendations for exertional dyspnea evaluation and EILO diagnosis presented in this review consider differences in perspective across continents and have incorporated feedback from providers across a variety of medical specialties (including generalists, allergists, pulmonologists, pediatricians, otolaryngologists, cardiologists, and sports medicine providers). Each of these perspectives is important because it is reasonable to hypothesize that providers of different backgrounds and specialties may differ in their experience with the presenting complaint, framework for considering the complaint, and interest in relevant differential diagnoses. Their experience may also vary with respect to their access to and experience with diagnostic testing and therapeutic interventions.

These recommendations incorporate those of consensus opinion panels convened to address the topic.[3,16] The review considers aspects of the presenting history with physical examination as well as the diagnostic work-up. Because the study of EILO is in its infancy when considered against exercise-induced asthma and exercise-induced bronchoconstriction (EIB), this article attempts to qualify recommendations with comments about literature strength in the area.

PRESENTATION AND HISTORY

Patients with EILO generally present with exertional dyspnea, although there is not a specific subset of symptoms that clearly defines a high likelihood of EILO, which has been validated across age, gender, race, ethnicity, and culture. Nonetheless, for decades, investigators have attempted to differentially characterize the prototypical symptoms in isolated EILO from those of patients with other conditions—especially isolated EILO.[17]

The concept of exercise-induced inspiratory symptoms (EIIS) has been used in the literature as an attempt to provide a label for the set of symptoms exhibited by patients with upper airway obstruction (**Fig. 1**).[18,19] EILO patients often qualitatively describe their dyspnea as a distressing "wheeze," something that occurred in 1 of the first publications on EILO,[4] despite that the prototypical EILO symptom is inspiratory stridor. Symptoms often occur during intense exercise, at times during episodes of exercise that are particularly important to the patient, and generally resolve within a few minutes.[17,20]

Patients may note that environmental conditions, especially temperature extremes, are associated with increasing likelihood of symptoms.[4] In describing EIIS, some investigators have noted descriptions of pain in the chest or throat area as well as associated hyperventilation.[21] Sometimes this pattern progresses to frank panic reactions, evolving in parallel with increasing ventilatory requirements as the intensity of the exercise increases.[22,23] The timing of symptoms (within the respiratory cycle, within a given exercise session, and with respect to recovery) is of critical importance when distinguishing EILO from asthma, with EILO symptoms typically starting in association with very intense exercise and resolving within a few minutes of exercise termination.[24]

In contrast, many patients with exercise-induced bronchospasm with asthma present with a long-standing history of known asthma.[25] Rather than describing discrete events with a clear beginning and end, these patients often describe shortness of breath with an onset after prolonged exercise and resolution remote from exercise

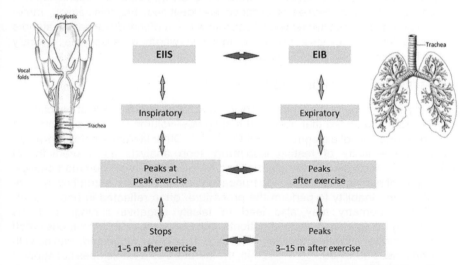

Fig. 1. Characteristics of EIIS versus symptoms of EIB. (*From* Røksund OD, Heimdal JH, Clemm H, et al. Exercise inducible laryngeal obstruction: diagnostics and management. Paediatr Respir Rev 2017;21:87; with permission.)

termination.[26,27] Cough is frequently associated, as is chest tightness. Audible respiration is often not perceived.[20] In the authors' experience, distress is frequently not described with the exception of severe events.

In the authors' experience, patients with exertional dyspnea, especially adolescents, sometimes struggle to fully characterize their symptoms at an initial visit. Some present with a vague sense of breathing problems that occur in relation to exercise, feeling unable to breathe and not "get enough air," particularly during intense exercise. Characterizing dyspnea within the respiratory cycle can be challenging, particularly for patients with expiratory limitation. One of the initial challenges faced by clinicians working with patients with exertional dyspnea is establishing a characteristic history without the use of excessively leading questions.

The clinical history may be more complicated to disentangle in reality than the impression conveyed in **Fig. 1**, which is presented as a way of distinguishing prototypical descriptions of EILO and EIB. Some of the prototypical descriptions of EILO may be based on the findings in seminal literature, which did not rely on direct visualization for diagnosis.[20,28,29] This approach also intentionally looks past other diseases that affect the cardiorespiratory system. As a clinician, it is important to acknowledge that there may be multiple phenotypes of both EIB and EILO, each with slightly different patient descriptions of symptoms. It is also important to consider that EILO and EIB may coexist, clouding the presentation.[5,10,17,20,28,30]

DIAGNOSTIC EVALUATION OF EXERTIONAL DYSPNEA WITH A FOCUS ON EXERCISE-INDUCED LARYNGEAL OBSTRUCTION

The authors agree with recent literature[3,19] and strongly recommend reserving a diagnosis of EILO for cases supported with direct visualization during characteristic events (as opposed to relying only on patients' histories or responses to therapeutic trials).[29,31] This advice is in line with published diagnostic recommendations for EIB.[25] This opinion is supported by diagnostic algorithms developed for military personnel in whom misinterpreting respiratory symptoms can be fatal.[32]

The likelihood of an EILO diagnosis varies, however, with clinical presentation and likely changes as other causes of dyspnea are identified. For this reason, rather than recommending definitive testing all patients with exertional dyspnea, the authors recommend limiting definitive testing to those in whom a reasonable clinically assessed pretest probability of EILO exists.

SPIROMETRY AND BRONCHOPROVOCATION TESTS

Spirometry is commonly available to providers across several medical specialties. Early literature suggested that abnormal resting flow-volume loops in patients with EIIS were suggestive of a diagnosis of EILO.[4,14,20,28] Other literature notes, however, suboptimal specificity of resting inspiratory loop analysis as a predictor of EILO.[20,28,33,34] According to Christopher and Morris,[22] the most common causes, for example, of resting inspiratory loop truncation are inadequate instruction, suboptimal effort, and inability to perform the procedure, often reflected in poor repeatability.[35,36] Spirometry may also lead to falsely negative findings and the sensitivity regarding identification of patients with EIIS is low.[7,20,28,33] Various cutoff levels for inspiratory versus expiratory flow ratios have been suggested, with no validated consensus obtained.[14,20,33,37] Thus, the literature as a whole does not support the notion that EILO can be confirmed or rejected by resting spirometry.

Spirometry is nevertheless important in patients with EIIS because it is central to the evaluation of asthma, subglottic stenosis, airway malacia, or intrathoracic compressions of various forms. Spirometry is also useful in the assessment of other chronic diseases. Distinct and fixed flattening of the inspiratory and/or expiratory parts of the flow-volume loops in patients with EIIS should incite further assessment.[22]

Spirometry can be combined with direct and indirect bronchoprovocation challenges in the assessment of asthma, but these challenges do not provoke characteristic events of EILO. It has been shown that bronchoprovocation challenges with either a methacholine or mannitol did not correlate with EILO as detected via continuous laryngoscopy during exercise (CLE test).[38] Most investigators have concluded that methacholine challenge tests are of little value to distinguish EILO from asthma, particularly because the 2 conditions are not mutually exclusive.[20,22,28,39] Spirometry during exercise, using exercise flow-volume loops, has been considered a potential diagnostic modality for EILO. Theoretic benefits of the modality include the noninvasive nature of the technique. At the current time, the technique has not been validated nor have threshold criteria been set to define the condition. It is unlikely that exercise flow-volume moves will become sufficient for the diagnosis of EILO for reasons related to interpretation of the test. Flow-volume loops change dramatically over the course of incremental exercise. Additionally, there are reports of patients with normal exercise flow-volume loops occurring simultaneous to symptoms, audible stridor, and the visualized findings of EILO.[40]

Currently, there is no evidence to suggest that other noninvasive techniques are useful to positively confirm diagnoses of EILO. Although impulse oscillometry has been hypothesized as having a potential role in the evaluation of exertional dyspnea in select cases, to the authors' knowledge, there has never been a case of EILO specifically diagnosed by impulse oscillometry.[41–43]

RESTING LARYNGOSCOPY

Although resting laryngoscopy can detect many upper airway lesions that are present at rest, there is not a role for this procedure in the definitive diagnosis of EILO because the changes seen in EILO are simply not present at rest.[23,24]

EXERCISE LARYNGOSCOPY

In the past few decades, postexercise (or a combination of prexercise and postexercise) laryngoscopy has been reported as a potential diagnostic technique for EILO.[44] Although this procedure can be performed in many settings and can detect EILO in some cases, sensitivity of the procedure is not ideal given the inherent time delay between exercise termination and larngoscope placement, even in the most ideal circumstances.[18,24]

CONTINUOUS LARYNGOSCOPY DURING EXERCISE

CLE is a procedure that allows laryngeal visualization via a held or fixed laryngoscope before, during, and after exercise.[23] The method has been described as easy to perform and well tolerated at centers with experience, even in young children.[18,19,45] CLE has been featured in several recent publications.[5,6,8,18–20,28,45–50] There are clearly logistic challenges to performing the procedure from a technical perspective. There are incremental improvements, however, in image acquisition compared with resting and postexercise laryngoscopy, specifically related to linking data acquisition to the exact time of symptom generation. A task force representing the European Respiratory Society (ERS), the European Laryngological Society (ELS), and the American College of Chest Physicians (ACCP), recently published a consensus document related to diagnostic considerations in ILO from all causes, including EILO.[3] In this document, a central principle in ILO diagnosis involves visualization during an episode of ILO. For this reason, CLE is identified as the preferred diagnostic technique for EILO. The suggested role played by CLE in the work-up of EIIS is depicted in **Fig. 2.**

PROCEDURAL CONSIDERATIONS

As a minimum requirement, a laryngoscope should be in place throughout the complete exercise session, which should be designed to reproduce characteristic field

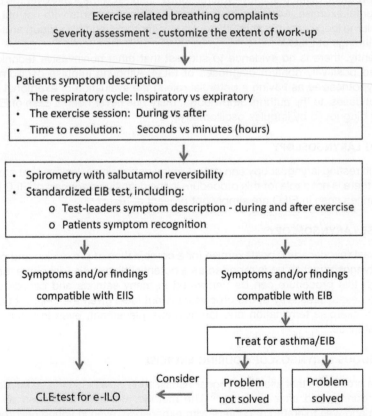

Fig. 2. Work-up should be customized to the level of complaints but should always involve a thorough symptom description. Spirometry, salbutamol reversibility, and a standardized test for EIB are logical second steps. The EIB test should always include a respiratory technician's description of breathing patterns and symptoms during and after the test and a patient verification that the symptoms perceived during the test were similar to those that incited the work-up. EIIS during testing without findings in the larynx must incite further work-up. (*From* Røksund OD, Heimdal JH, Clemm H, et al. Exercise inducible laryngeal obstruction: diagnostics and management. Paediatr Respir Rev 2017;21:88; with permission.)

symptoms as defined by the patient. The findings can be recorded for documentation and later review and analysis. A CLE setup can easily be combined with synchronized acquisition of cardiopulmonary exercise data and external video and breath sound recordings of the patient that can then be merged into 1 digitalized file.[23]

Exercise Mode

When performing CLE, selection of an exercise mode is an important consideration. Treadmill running, ergometer cycling, rowing, stair climbing, and swimming have all been used to reproduce EIIS in a diagnostic setting.[20,23,46,49,51–53] Ideally, the mode, protocol, and intensity of exercise should be tailored to the individual patient, based on triggers identified from the medical history, as described in rowers by Panchasara and colleagues[52] and in swimmers by Walsted and colleagues.[53] In routine clinics, there must be compromise but at minimum ensuring that exercise continues to exhaustion or to intolerable symptoms. In most young people, treadmill exercise is a more provocative respiratory stimulus than cycle ergometry.[54] Tervonen and colleagues[46] used a stationary bicycle and were unable to reproduce symptoms in 50% of patients with EIIS and made laryngeal findings in 30%. Some of the inherent environmental limitations present in hospital settings could be overcome by field testing. Although conceptually possible, field testing for EILO has not yet been reported from studies.

Protocol Considerations

In most publications featuring CLE, incremental exercise protocols have been used to generate symptoms.[24,46] Incremental exercise protocols are popular in a variety of fields of medicine, in part because they allow for the reproduction of metabolic data in a fairly standardized way across patients. More recently, a high-intensity interval protocol was reported.[24] There is no evidence that incremental protocols provide the most provocative respiratory stimulus compared with other protocols with respect to EILO. Although tempting to combine the procedure with provocative challenges for asthma, it is important to consider that EILO and EIB are different conditions, presumably involving different causal mechanisms. For this reason, it is unlikely that the same provocative trigger is most effective for both EILO and EIB.

Data Interpretation: What Is Normal?

During exercise, the larynx normally opens fully and the epiglottis rotates anteriorly toward the base of the tongue,[49] stretching the aryepiglottic folds, thereby allowing for increased airflow with least possible increase of airflow resistance.[48] The posterior cricoarytenoid muscle is the only laryngeal abductor, acting in a synchronized manner with and ahead of the diaphragm, ensuring that the laryngeal entrance is wide open when inspiratory airflow commences.[55–57] Few patients have been studied with the aim of characterizing in detail what should be considered normal laryngeal configuration at peak ventilation. Some data suggest that a slight adduction of the aryepiglottic folds at peak ventilation is normal.[18,49]

Anatomic Descriptions of Exercise-Induced Laryngeal Obstruction

The anatomy, physiology, nervous regulation, and function of the larynx are complex matters, and corresponding heterogeneities in reported findings are expected. In the largest study of EIIS to date, 151 patients were CLE tested with findings compatible with EILO in 113 (75%).[18] Adduction started at a supraglottic level in 109, with later glottic involvement in 88. Medialization of the vocal folds generally was noted anteriorly. Primary glottic adduction was rare. Corresponding data are reported also by other investigators.[5,6,8,19,58]

Thresholds of Disease

The specific changes in airflow or the laryngeal aperture that define disease have not been physiologically validated. Regarding the vocal gap, McFadden and Zawadski[28] proposed that an adduction exceeding 50% was consistent with EILO. Other investigators have defined EILO in terms of semiquantitative scaling.[18] Importantly, most of the airflow through larynx normally takes place in the dorsal part of the glottic aperture, which is the part initially obstructed by medializing aryepiglottic folds.[18]

Reporting Findings

The recent ERS/ELS/ACCP task force report[3] requests continuous laryngoscopy to be performed from rest to peak exercise and visual verification of adducting laryngeal structures occurring concomitant to symptoms to assign a diagnosis of EILO to a patient.[3] The taxonomy differentiates between 2 categories of EILO—glottic and a supraglottic—and acknowledges that these categories can appear separately or combined. Combined glottic and supraglottic EILO may not be cotemporal throughout an attack, and the taxonomy requests each component be separately described and their temporal relation detailed. These distinctions are certainly of practical importance, because patients with severe collapse of supraglottic structures can be treated by laser supraglottoplasty.[59–62] These distinctions also lead to realizations that terminology that isolates disease to the level of the glottis (vocal cord dysfunction and paradoxic vocal fold motion) is outdated.[29,63,64]

Why Has Continuous Laryngoscopy During Exercise Been Slowly Integrated into Clinical Care?

Christopher and Morris[22] showed in their review from 2010 that laryngoscopy had not been performed in 38% of 355 assessed articles on ILO (not all exercise induced), with CLE rarely used in the studies cited. There are many factors that may explain some of the reluctance of clinicians and researchers in adopting the testing modality. First, the diagnostic yield reported from studies applying the principles of the CLE in patients with EIIS has varied.[10,18,46] This may be related to the fact that there is likely heterogeneity across populations in terms of the frequency of EIIS, the proportion of subjects with EIIS struggling with EILO, the expertise of referral centers, and differences in testing environments, protocols, and data interpretation. Second, logistic considerations with regards to space, personnel, and resources may be a deterrent.

AREAS FOR FUTURE GROWTH

Although CLE offers several advantages over other forms of diagnostic testing for EILO, there are still several opportunities for future improvement. There is currently no consensus on testing protocols. There is also no consensus on the findings that define disease, which may vary with body habitus, gender, fitness, or athletic level. Current laryngoscopy analysis is subjective and restricted to relative assessments of the cross-sectional laryngeal size, because this changes from rest to peak exercise. A notable gap in scientific knowledge relates to the poor understanding of normal laryngeal size and function in absolute terms and in relation to features, such as gender, body habitus, physical fitness, and exercise capacity. For example, a similar extent of adduction is likely to have different consequences in a narrow larynx compared with a wide larynx and also in a competing athlete compared with a sedentary person. Linking laryngoscopy with physiologic data, including pressure gradients, may help define the importance of current laryngoscopy observations of unclear significance.

SUMMARY

EILO is one cause of EIIS and it is an important diagnosis due to its high prevalence and the ability to treat the condition. It is not reasonable to rely on the clinical history alone, flow-volume loops, or resting laryngoscopy to define the condition. CLE offers notable advantages over postexercise laryngoscopy in terms of diagnosing EILO. Many facility-specific logistic challenges and questions regarding the interpretation of the data have, however, limited its wide-scale use to date.

REFERENCES

1. Abu-Hasan M, Tannous B, Weinberger M. Exercise-induced dyspnea in children and adolescents: if not asthma then what? Ann Allergy Asthma Immunol 2005; 94(3):366–71.
2. Hurbis CG, Schild JA. Laryngeal changes during exercise and exercise-induced asthma. Ann Otol Rhinol Laryngol 1991;100(1):34–7.
3. Christensen PM, Heimdal JH, Christopher KL, et al. ERS/ELS/ACCP 2013 international consensus conference nomenclature on inducible laryngeal obstructions. Eur Respir Rev 2015;24(137):445–50.
4. Lakin RC, Metzger WJ, Haughey BH. Upper airway obstruction presenting as exercise-induced asthma. Chest 1984;86(3):499–501.
5. Johansson H, Norlander K, Berglund L, et al. Prevalence of exercise-induced bronchoconstriction and exercise-induced laryngeal obstruction in a general adolescent population. Thorax 2015;70(1):57–63.
6. Christensen PM, Thomsen SF, Rasmussen N, et al. Exercise-induced laryngeal obstructions: prevalence and symptoms in the general public. Eur Arch Otorhinolaryngol 2011;268(9):1313–9.
7. Morris MJ, Deal LE, Bean DR, et al. Vocal cord dysfunction in patients with exertional dyspnea. Chest 1999;116(6):1676–82.
8. Nielsen EW, Hull JH, Backer V. High prevalence of exercise-induced laryngeal obstruction in athletes. Med Sci Sports Exerc 2013;45(11):2030–5.
9. Garber CE, Blissmer B, Deschenes MR, et al. American College of Sports Medicine position stand. Quantity and quality of exercise for developing and maintaining cardiorespiratory, musculoskeletal, and neuromotor fitness in apparently healthy adults: guidance for prescribing exercise. Med Sci Sports Exerc 2011; 43(7):1334–59.
10. Newman KB, Mason UG III, Schmaling KB. Clinical features of vocal cord dysfunction. Am J Respir Crit Care Med 1995;152(4 Pt 1):1382–6.
11. Keeley DJ, Silverman M. Issues at the interface between primary and secondary care in the management of common respiratory disease.2: Are we too ready to diagnose asthma in children? Thorax 1999;54(7):625–8.
12. Asthma inhalers handed out like fashion accessories, doctors warn. The Telegraph (United Kingdom). April 5, 2016.
13. Patterson R, Schatz M, Horton M. Munchausen's stridor: non-organic laryngeal obstruction. Clin Allergy 1974;4(3):307–10.
14. Christopher KL, Wood RP, Eckert RC, et al. Vocal-cord dysfunction presenting as asthma. N Engl J Med 1983;308(26):1566–70.

15. Selner JC, Staudenmayer H, Koepke JW, et al. Vocal cord dysfunction: the importance of psychologic factors and provocation challenge testing. J Allergy Clin Immunol 1987;79(5):726–33.
16. Halvorsen T, Schwarz Walsted E, Bucca C, et al. Inducible laryngeal obstruction: an official joint European Respiratory Society and European Laryngological Society statement. Eur Respir J 2017;50(3) [pii:1602221].
17. Landwehr LP, Wood RP, Blager FB, et al. Vocal cord dysfunction mimicking exercise-induced bronchospasm in adolescents. Pediatrics 1996;98(5):971–4.
18. Roksund OD, Maat RC, Heimdal JH, et al. Exercise induced dyspnea in the young. Larynx as the bottleneck of the airways. Respir Med 2009;103(12): 1911–8.
19. Buchvald F, Phillipsen LD, Hjuler T, et al. Exercise-induced inspiratory symptoms in school children. Pediatr Pulmonol 2016;51(11):1200–5.
20. Rundell KW, Spiering BA. Inspiratory stridor in elite athletes. Chest 2003;123(2): 468–74.
21. Roksund OD, Heimdal JH, Clemm H, et al. Exercise inducible laryngeal obstruction: diagnostics and management. Paediatr Respir Rev 2017;21:86–94.
22. Christopher KL, Morris MJ. Vocal cord dysfunction, paradoxic vocal fold motion, or laryngomalacia? Our understanding requires an interdisciplinary approach. Otolaryngol Clin North Am 2010;43(1):43–66, viii.
23. Heimdal JH, Roksund OD, Halvorsen T, et al. Continuous laryngoscopy exercise test: a method for visualizing laryngeal dysfunction during exercise. Laryngoscope 2006;116(1):52–7.
24. Olin JT, Clary MS, Fan EM, et al. Continuous laryngoscopy quantitates laryngeal behaviour in exercise and recovery. Eur Respir J 2016;48(4):1192–200.
25. Parsons JP, Hallstrand TS, Mastronarde JG, et al. An official American Thoracic Society clinical practice guideline: exercise-induced bronchoconstriction. Am J Respir Crit Care Med 2013;187(9):1016–27.
26. Kattan M, Keens TG, Mellis CM, et al. The response to exercise in normal and asthmatic children. J Pediatr 1978;92(5):718–21.
27. Hofstra WB, Sterk PJ, Neijens HJ, et al. Prolonged recovery from exercise-induced asthma with increasing age in childhood. Pediatr Pulmonol 1995;20(3): 177–83.
28. McFadden ER Jr, Zawadski DK. Vocal cord dysfunction masquerading as exercise-induced asthma. a physiologic cause for "choking" during athletic activities. Am J Respir Crit Care Med 1996;153(3):942–7.
29. Maturo S, Hill C, Bunting G, et al. Pediatric paradoxical vocal-fold motion: presentation and natural history. Pediatrics 2011;128(6):e1443–9.
30. Wilson JJ, Wilson EM. Practical management: vocal cord dysfunction in athletes. Clin J Sport Med 2006;16(4):357–60.
31. Krafczyk MA, Asplund CA. Exercise-induced bronchoconstriction: diagnosis and management. Am Fam Physician 2011;84(4):427–34.
32. Morris MJ, Lucero PF, Zanders TB, et al. Diagnosis and management of chronic lung disease in deployed military personnel. Ther Adv Respir Dis 2013;7(4): 235–45.
33. Christensen PM, Maltbaek N, Jorgensen IM, et al. Can flow-volume loops be used to diagnose exercise induced laryngeal obstructions? A comparison study examining the accuracy and inter-rater agreement of flow volume loops as a diagnostic tool. Prim Care Respir J 2013;22(3):306–11.
34. Morrison M, Rammage L, Emami AJ. The irritable larynx syndrome. J Voice 1999; 13(3):447–55.

35. Ruppel GL. The inspiratory flow-volume curve: the neglected child of pulmonary diagnostics. Respir Care 2009;54(4):448–9.
36. Sterner JB, Morris MJ, Sill JM, et al. Inspiratory flow-volume curve evaluation for detecting upper airway disease. Respir Care 2009;54(4):461–6.
37. Kenn K, Balkissoon R. Vocal cord dysfunction: what do we know? Eur Respir J 2011;37(1):194–200.
38. Walsted ES, Hull JH, Sverrild A, et al. Bronchial provocation testing does not detect exercise-induced laryngeal obstruction. J Asthma 2017;54(1):77–83.
39. Brugman SM, Simons SM. Vocal cord dysfunction: don't mistake it for asthma. Phys Sportsmed 1998;26(5):63–85.
40. Olin JT, Clary MS, Connors D, et al. Glottic configuration in patients with exercise-induced stridor: a new paradigm. Laryngoscope 2014;124(11):2568–73.
41. Malmberg LP, Makela MJ, Mattila PS, et al. Exercise-induced changes in respiratory impedance in young wheezy children and nonatopic controls. Pediatr Pulmonol 2008;43(6):538–44.
42. Price OJ, Ansley L, Bikov A, et al. The role of impulse oscillometry in detecting airway dysfunction in athletes. J Asthma 2016;53(1):62–8.
43. Komarow HD, Young M, Nelson C, et al. Vocal cord dysfunction as demonstrated by impulse oscillometry. J Allergy Clin Immunol Pract 2013;1(4):387–93.
44. Chiang T, Marcinow AM, deSilva BW, et al. Exercise-induced paradoxical vocal fold motion disorder: diagnosis and management. Laryngoscope 2013;123(3): 727–31.
45. Sidell DR, Balakrishnan K, Hart CK, et al. Pediatric exercise stress laryngoscopy following laryngotracheoplasty: a comparative review. Otolaryngol Head Neck Surg 2014;150(6):1056–61.
46. Tervonen H, Niskanen MM, Sovijarvi AR, et al. Fiberoptic videolaryngoscopy during bicycle ergometry: a diagnostic tool for exercise-induced vocal cord dysfunction. Laryngoscope 2009;119(9):1776–80.
47. Tilles SA, Inglis AF. Masqueraders of exercise-induced vocal cord dysfunction. J Allergy Clin Immunol 2009;124(2):377–8, 78.
48. Beaty MM, Wilson JS, Smith RJ. Laryngeal motion during exercise. Laryngoscope 1999;109(1):136–9.
49. Bent JP III, Miller DA, Kim JW, et al. Pediatric exercise-induced laryngomalacia. Ann Otol Rhinol Laryngol 1996;105(3):169–75.
50. Ibrahim WH, Gheriani HA, Almohamed AA, et al. Paradoxical vocal cord motion disorder: past, present and future. Postgrad Med J 2007;83(977):164–72.
51. Christopher KL. Understanding vocal cord dysfunction: a step in the right direction with a long road ahead. Chest 2006;129(4):842–3.
52. Panchasara B, Nelson C, Niven R, et al. Lesson of the month: rowing-induced laryngeal obstruction: a novel cause of exertional dyspnoea: characterised by direct laryngoscopy. Thorax 2015;70(1):95–7.
53. Walsted ES, Swanton LL, van van Someren K, et al. Laryngoscopy during swimming: a novel diagnostic technique to characterize swimming- induced laryngeal obstruction. Laryngoscope 2017. https://doi.org/10.1002/lary.26532.
54. Åstrand PO, RK, Dahl HA, et al. Physical performance; Evaluation of physical performance on the basis of tests. In: Textbook of work physiology. Physiological bases of exercise. 4th edition. Stockholm (Sweden): Human Kinetics; 2003. p. 237–99.
55. Belmont JR, Grundfast K, Rodahl K. Congenital laryngeal stridor (laryngomalacia). In: Bahrke MS. etiologic factors and associated disorders. Ann Otol Rhinol Laryngol 1984;93(5 Pt 1):430–7.

56. Brancatisano TP, Dodd DS, Engel LA. Respiratory activity of posterior cricoarytenoid muscle and vocal cords in humans. J Appl Physiol Respir Environ Exerc Physiol 1984;57(4):1143–9.

57. Petcu LG, Sasaki CT. Laryngeal anatomy and physiology. Clin Chest Med 1991; 12(3):415–23.

58. Nordang L, Moren S, Johansson HM, et al. Exercise-induced asthma could be laryngeal obstruction. Not uncommon among young sportsmen–avoiding the wrong treatment is important. Lakartidningen 2009;106(38):2351–3 [in Swedish].

59. Maat RC, Roksund OD, Olofsson J, et al. Surgical treatment of exercise-induced laryngeal dysfunction. Eur Arch Otorhinolaryngol 2007;264(4):401–7.

60. Maat RC, Hilland M, Roksund OD, et al. Exercise-induced laryngeal obstruction: natural history and effect of surgical treatment. Eur Arch Otorhinolaryngol 2011; 268(10):1485–92.

61. Norlander K, Johansson H, Jansson C, et al. Surgical treatment is effective in severe cases of exercise-induced laryngeal obstruction: a follow-up study. Acta Otolaryngol 2015;135(11):1152–9.

62. Mehlum CS, Walsted ES, Godballe C, et al. Supraglottoplasty as treatment of exercise induced laryngeal obstruction (EILO). Eur Arch Otorhinolaryngol 2016; 273(4):945–51.

63. Turmel J, Gagnon S, Bernier M, et al. Eucapnic voluntary hyperpnoea and exercise-induced vocal cord dysfunction. BMJ Open Sport Exerc Med 2015; 1(1):e000065.

64. Palla J, Friedman AD. Paradoxical vocal cord motion in pediatric patients. Pediatr Ann 2016;45(5):e184–8.

Speech-Language Pathology as a Primary Treatment for Exercise-Induced Laryngeal Obstruction

Monica Shaffer, MA, CCC-SLP[a],*, Juliana K. Litts, MA, CCC-SLP[b],
Emily Nauman, MA, CCC-SLP[a], Jemma Haines, CertMRCSLT[c]

KEYWORDS

- Speech-language pathology (SLP) • Exercise-induced laryngeal obstruction (EILO)
- Paradoxical vocal fold motion (PVFM) • Vocal cord dysfunction (VCD)
- Pursed lip breathing • Laryngeal control therapy

KEY POINTS

- Exercise-induced laryngeal obstruction responds well to behavioral therapy guided by a speech-language pathologist.
- Traditional therapy techniques include education, relaxation, and instruction on various breathing techniques, such as pursed lip breathing or sniffing.
- Paced exercise with applied breathing techniques can prevent and alleviate symptoms of exercise-induced laryngeal obstruction.
- Many individuals experience near full resolution of exercise-induced laryngeal obstruction symptoms with traditional therapy techniques, although there are refractory cases requiring additional intervention approaches.

INTRODUCTION

Exercise-induced laryngeal obstruction (EILO) is a pattern of glottic and/or supraglottic closure that restricts an individual's ability to inhale and exhale comfortably in response to exercise. Historically, EILO has been identified by many names such as vocal cord dysfunction or paradoxical vocal fold motion.

Disclosure Statement: No relevant financial nor nonfinancial relationships exist for all contributing authors.
[a] Rehab Department, National Jewish Health, 1400 Jackson Street, Denver, CO 80206, USA;
[b] Department of Otolaryngology, University of Colorado Hospital, 12631 East 17th Avenue, B-205, Aurora, CO 80045, USA; [c] Department of Respiratory Medicine, North West Lung Centre, Wythenshawe Hospital, Manchester University National Health Service Foundation Trust, Southmoor Road, Manchester, M23 9LT, UK
* Corresponding author.
E-mail address: Shafferm@njhealth.org

Regarding treatment, EILO responds well to behavioral therapy and respiratory retraining. Since it was first described in the nonpsychiatric literature, speech-language pathologists (SLPs) have been involved in the assessment and treatment of patients with EILO.[1] SLPs are formally trained in the assessment and treatment of disorders of the aerodigestive tract and facilitating behavioral change via patient education, relaxation, and respiratory retraining. In treating EILO, SLPs use various approaches of breathing and relaxation techniques to guide the patient through symptom prevention, control, and rescue breathing during their dyspneic episodes. The literature suggests positive patient response to behavioral intervention for EILO.[1–14] It has been reported that behavioral intervention by SLPs may prevent up to 90% of patient visits to the emergency room for symptoms attributable to inducible laryngeal obstruction, although this finding is not specific to patients with exercise-induced symptoms.[15]

In this review, guidelines for treatment approaches in patients with EILO using behavioral interventions are outlined. Traditional approaches to therapy are discussed, as well as additional interventions for refractory EILO, and future directions for research and therapy.

TREATMENT OVERVIEW

Speech-language intervention for EILO is a short course of guided therapy (2–3 sessions) by SLPs specializing in voice and respiratory disorders. Treatment involves various approaches and should be tailored to the patient. Traditional treatment approaches include patient education, patient counseling, relaxation techniques, and training in specific breathing techniques that optimize laryngeal relaxation, respiratory pace, and patient comfort. Medical interventions for comorbid diagnoses should also be considered by the referring doctor and may include treatment for asthma, sinonasal disease, laryngopharyngeal reflux, allergic rhinitis, and anxiety.

Education and Reassurance

The first goal of treatment is educating the patient on their diagnosis and goals of therapy.[10,12–14,16,17] Often, patients are frustrated and confused by the time a correct diagnosis and treatment plan is established, because EILO is commonly misdiagnosed.[18,19] It is our experience that many adolescent athletes with EILO are not allowed to participate in competitive sports given observer fear of noisy laryngeal stridor. The treating SLP plays an important role in educating the patient and those involved in the patient's activity or sport of choice (including coaches, teachers, and parents). Reassurance that EILO is not life threatening helps to alleviate fear for both the patient and observers.[6,12]

It is our experience that patient understanding of laryngeal anatomy and physiology aids the patient in independent symptom control. If available, images from the patient's diagnostic laryngoscopy may be used to enhance patient understanding.[9,12,20] Alternatively, laryngeal models or artist depictions of the anatomy are useful teaching tools.[21] It is our experience that patients benefit through learning relevant respiratory physiology. Keys to anatomic/physiologic teaching are summarized in **Table 1**.

Helping patients to characterize and describe their symptoms is important for the prevention and control of dyspneic episodes. It is our experience that the sooner patients can identify the initial onset of symptoms during exercise, the easier the symptoms are to control. Simple questions to stimulate this conversation with a patient are summarized in **Table 2**. Along with anatomy and physiology teaching, it is also important to teach safety with patients who may have more severe episodes (**Box 1**).

Table 1	
Key teaching points for patient education	
Teaching Point	**Description**
Anatomic	Vocal cords sit on top of the trachea and lungs
Physiologic	Normal vocal cord movement: open with breathing, close with speech for vibration, close for protective behaviors (coughing, throat clearing, breathholding)
	Biological function of the vocal folds is protective; coughing and throat clearing are behaviors to eject irritants from the larynx and require vocal cord closure
	Vocal cords are built to open with air pressure from the lungs below; this is how voice is produced
Respiratory physiology	Rapidly moving air through a restricted area (larynx) can produce turbulence, causing a sensation of restricted airflow
	If the patient has spirometry demonstrating truncated inspiratory flow, discuss how the larynx or pharynx may be contributing to this
EILO specifics	Speed of inspiratory or expiratory airflow can be irritating to a hypersensitive system and can precipitate or prolong the symptoms of EILO
	Bring the patient's attention to importance of breath out, as well as the breath in, which is not intuitive when patient is feeling symptoms of dyspnea
	Patients with dyspnea during exercise often cause worsened symptoms by not allowing enough time for a full exhale to empty lungs and allow for complete inspiration
	Impart idea of patient control over respiratory and laryngeal mechanisms

Abbreviation: EILO, exercise-induced laryngeal obstruction.

Traditional Rescue Breathing: Pursed Lip Breathing and Laryngeal Control Therapy

Traditional modes of treatment for EILO aim to adjust oropharyngolaryngeal aperture during exercise and symptomatic episodes via various breathing and relaxation techniques, often grouped under the term "laryngeal control therapy."[2] Effective treatment

Table 2	
Questions to establish description and characterization of EILO symptoms	
Questions	**Rationale**
What specific activities, sports, and exertional levels trigger your episodes?	If a patient engages in multiple sports, one may be more bothersome to EILO symptoms than others.
Can you predict when you are going to have an episode? What do you feel leading up to the episode?	Initial symptom presentation is described differently between patients. Establish language with the patient to understand and identify these early symptoms.
How quickly do symptoms begin when you start exercising? How quickly do symptoms resolve when you stop exercise?	Characterizing bouts in the context of exercise timeframe will allow the patient to better predict onset, and to better pace exercise based on symptom severity.
What do you do to make the episode better?	Using appropriate strategies devised by the patient may further therapeutic progress. It may be necessary to educate patient on avoiding inappropriate strategies (eg, hyperventilating).

Abbreviation: EILO, exercise-induced laryngeal obstruction.

> **Box 1**
> **Educating safety in patients with severe EILO**
>
> EILO will not cause death by asphyxiation.
>
> With loss of consciousness, respiratory patterns will return to normal, although loss of consciousness is a greater safety hazard in certain sports (eg, swimming).
>
> When feeling lightheaded or dyspneic, stop operating heavy machinery (eg, car), sit down in a safe location without objects that could cause injury (eg, coffee table, book shelf, stairs, etc).
>
> Attempt to use some breathing techniques, as instructed in therapy, to regain control of respiratory system.
>
> If an ER visit is necessary, develop a plan for communication to the ER providers; avoid extreme measures for EILO treatment, such as tracheotomy, in favor of other interventions such as heliox.
>
> *Abbreviations*: EILO, exercise-induced laryngeal obstruction; ER, emergency room.

is tailored to each patient based on clinical discussions and the patient's symptom severity ratings when using various techniques. Specific breathing techniques that may be used are described herein; primary approaches and their initial publication are summarized in **Table 3**.

First described by Christopher and colleagues (1983),[1] pursed lip breathing is centered around giving the patient control over the breathing mechanism by producing restriction in the oral cavity during exhalation to match any laryngeal impedance during inhalation. Exhalation can be taught in a variety of different forms (**Table 4**).

Inhalation using a sniff technique (short and forceful nasal inhalation) has been suggested to maximize glottic opening.[5,16,21,22] Under laryngeal control therapy, Chiang and colleagues (2013)[2] suggested sniff inhalation with controlled exhalation as described. Other theories of respiratory retraining have emphasized the importance of silent inhalation that is relatively short (1–2 seconds) compared with the longer exhalation cycle.[12] This decreases the chance of prolonging the dyspnea episode owing to high-velocity air irritating the laryngeal mechanism.

A core foundational skill for EILO symptom management is diaphragmatic breathing, no matter what specific technique is being implemented. All approaches emphasize the importance of abdominal breathing, versus thoracic or clavicular patterns. With athletes in particular, an increased focus on lower rib excursion can prove more functional than a sole focus on abdominal breathing. This allows the patient to engage abdominal muscles for core support during exertion, while still using diaphragmatic breathing patterns. The mechanism through which diaphragmatic breathing may improve EILO is unclear at the current time.

Breathing techniques instructed in the clinic setting typically require adjustment for application during exercise, given the increased demand on the respiratory system. During exercise with high respiratory drive, it may not be possible or comfortable for the patient to breathe in through the nose, as with the sniff technique, or to use diaphragmatic breathing. Teaching pursed lip or oral inspiration may be necessary. It is important that the inspiratory phase of the breath cycle remains controlled and almost silent. The treating SLP should encourage the patient to find a mechanism of breath control that feels most comfortable for them, because there is no ubiquitous treatment that works for all patients.

At first onset of EILO symptoms, patients are instructed to implement a form of "release breathing." The patient may alternate between a more natural breathing

Table 3
Primary approaches to respiratory retraining

Approach/Technique	Description	Publication(s)
Laryngeal control therapy	• Focus on low abdominal movement • Audible nasal sniffing on inhalation • Controlled exhalation through the mouth with continuous or pulsed bursts via puckered lips • Goal is to improve awareness, perform slow breathing, and increase force on exhalation	Chiang et al,[2] 2013; Marcinow et al,[7] 2014
Pursed lip breathing	• Focus attention away from larynx and inspiration • Active expiration via abdominal muscles • Relaxed oropharyngeal muscle groups	Christopher et al,[1] 1983
Release breathing	• Focus on midabdominal movement with instruction to lower shoulders • Quick, 1-s inhale through nose or mouth • Exhale through tightly pursed lips for 2–3 s • Also provides strategies for cough and throat clearing elimination	Hicks et al,[16] 2008
Wide-open throat breathing or relaxed throat breathing	• Focus on openness and relaxation • Closed lips, tongue lies flat on floor of mouth behind lower front teeth, jaw is gently released • Use of diaphragm for inhalation and exhalation, with conscious attention away from laryngeal area • Also focuses on slow direction, increased self-awareness, and interruption of effortful breathing	Martin et al,[9] 1987

Table 4
Teaching exhalation

Approaches to exhalation	Short puffs of air through pursed lips like blowing out a candle repeatedly. Repeated bursts of voiceless sounds (s, f, sh) that are repeated 3–4 times before returning to inhalation. Long continuous exhalation through restriction with pursed lips. Continuous voiceless sounds (s, f, sh) lasting about 4 s. Exhalation through a straw held between the lips; however, this is not a functional option for most athletes.
Additional considerations	Degree of pursed lip opening is adjusted based on activity level and patient preference (eg, for running, a more rounded lip posture may be preferable, whereas a more tightly pursed posture is appropriate for walking or jogging) owing to presumed differences in the degree of laryngeal constriction between high respiratory drive in running vs walking. Metered exhalation during exercise or stair climbing with the patient experimenting with a rhythm for breathing that feels comfortable and controlled. For example, when climbing stairs, 4–5 steps for a breath out using a pursed lip technique and 2–3 steps for a breath in through nose. Different meters may be used for running vs walking.

pattern with a rounded lip exhale when asymptomatic, to a more pursed lip rescue breathing pattern when symptomatic. Resolution of symptoms should take less than 1 minute. In some cases, it is only necessary to do a few rescue breathing cycles before the symptoms abate. Lightheadedness can occur when the patient performs rescue breathing for a prolonged period of time. Slowing the pace of exertion at first onset of EILO symptoms can also help the patient to attend to their breath cycle and better resolve the episode. The patient may resume a faster pace of exertion and return to their more normal breathing pattern once symptoms have resolved. Learning appropriate pacing of exercise can be difficult for patients individually, and often therapeutic techniques have to be applied incrementally in a hierarchical structure with the SLP. Therefore, functional practice with the clinician present as the patient exercises in their preferred manner (eg, running, swimming, gymnastics, etc) will improve progress in therapy.[7,12,14] This practice can be challenging in a clinic setting without access to appropriate exercise equipment.

Recently, a new series of breathing techniques called the Olin EILOBI breathing techniques were described as a potential option for patients that remain symptomatic despite adequate performance of conventional respiratory retraining techniques during high-intensity exercise.[23] The principle behind these techniques is that sudden changes in airflow seem to positively affect inspiratory laryngeal configuration. The initial discovery of the techniques was largely visual and preliminary data suggest that these techniques are worthy of further study.[23,24]

Relaxation Techniques

In certain patients with EILO, excessive tension in the upper body, shoulders, neck, jaw, or face can contribute to worsened symptom severity in our experience. Improving patterns of diaphragmatic breathing is the first step in reducing excessive tension. Other techniques that help to relieve undue tightness are summarized in **Box 2**.

ADDITIONAL TREATMENT APPROACHES FOR REFRACTORY EXERCISE-INDUCED LARYNGEAL OBSTRUCTION

Many patients experience great benefit from traditional therapy approaches, with 75% to 80% experiencing improved or complete resolution of symptoms after respiratory

---

Box 2
Strategies for releasing excessive upper body tension

Instruction on voice therapy techniques of lip trills, tongue trills, or voiced sounds of /z, v, ʒ/.

Stretching targeted neck or shoulder muscles both in front and back to relieve tension.

Instruction on visualization of an open and relaxed airway. Referring back to laryngoscopy images may be helpful for certain patients.

Negative practice of creating a tight/closed feeling in their throat and then releasing muscles to create a more relaxed feeling.[10]

Verbally highlighting possible areas of tension and stress in shoulders and back of neck during exercises (eg, holding shoulders up while running); visual feedback via a mirror may be useful for some patients.

Instruction on breath awareness of difference between thoracic/clavicular breathing and abdominal breathing.

Instruction on avoidance of breathholding, which can frequently occur in activities such as weight lifting.

retraining.[2,25,26] However, there are patients for whom traditional approaches do not fully alleviate symptoms. The treating SLP may opt to implement additional tools for improvement in those patients that continue to struggle under traditional therapy approaches alone.

Inspiratory Muscle Training

Inspiratory muscle training (IMT) involves systematic periods of resistive breathing maneuvers designed to improve inspiratory muscle strength. Patients with EILO often present with symptoms including tachypnea as well as laborious breathing during periods of maximal exertion. These symptoms are similar in presentation to those with inspiratory muscle weakness.[27]

There have been numerous studies validating the role of IMT in patients with known respiratory impairments, in trained athletic populations and in typical, healthy aging adults.[27–33] Mathers-Schmidt and Brilla (2005)[11] revealed IMT improved inspiratory muscle strength and decreased a patient's overall exertional dyspnea rating in an 18-year-old female soccer player with EILO. In this study, the patient was initially provided traditional therapy techniques (education and relaxed throat breathing) before the implementation of an IMT protocol.

Biofeedback

The use of biofeedback has been demonstrated to improve patient control over the laryngeal mechanism.[2,3,6,7,20] It has been established that individuals can change laryngeal movements and postures using visual feedback of their own real-time laryngeal video as a learning tool.[34] Olin and colleagues (2016)[35] reported the first systematic use of therapeutic laryngoscopy during exercise (TLE) in individuals with EILO refractory to treatment, despite receiving a range of behavioral therapies. During TLE, EILO symptoms are provoked. This process allows individuals and clinicians to visualize, tailor therapy, and apply techniques incrementally to improve laryngeal aperture in real-time. Olin and colleagues (2016)[35] reported that three-quarters of participants agreed or strongly agreed that their breathing during exercise had improved with TLE and, of those participants, 85% felt TLE was the most important therapy leading to breathing improvement.

Heliox

Heliox is a mixture of helium and oxygen, which has no bronchodilating nor antiinflammatory properties and can be used safely in most individuals.[36] Compared with room air and oxygen, heliox has different laminar flow characteristics.[37] Its lower density means that it can pass through partial upper airway obstruction with ease,[38] reducing turbulent airflow[39] and facilitating better free-flowing laminar flow. The resulting reduction in airway resistance[40] decreases the individual's sense of dyspnea and effort.[36]

Although heliox has been reported as efficacious in the treatment of acute episodes of upper airway obstruction,[41] administration concurrently with exercise is an unlikely approach owing to the prescribed mode of delivery: 5 to 10 minutes through a nonrebreather facemask until symptoms resolve.[37] Heliox maybe more appropriately used as a tool to aid quicker recovery of an EILO attack and facilitate return to a high respiratory drive in competitive events. Further investigation and research are required to understand the use of heliox in EILO management. Randomized, blinded, and controlled prospective research is necessary to determine the true therapeutic potential of this treatment.

FUTURE CONSIDERATIONS

Much of the currently available literature is composed of case studies, retrospective chart reviews, or descriptive articles outlining the signs and symptoms of EILO. High-quality research studies on specific treatment approaches are needed to improve our understanding of this disorder to fully ascertain if complete resolution of symptoms across all patients is achievable. Additionally, although recreational athletes are generally able to manage symptoms via traditional therapy approaches and paced exercise, it is our experience that high-performance athletes may experience more refractory symptoms. For professional athletes or highly competitive athletes, a slower pace for symptom resolution is often not an option. Research of additional breathing techniques for high-performance athletes or maximum-level exertion is needed as an alternative for this population.

SUMMARY

SLPs have been shown to be appropriate providers to facilitate behavioral change and patient control over EILO symptoms. Further research is needed to understand the mechanism of SLP intervention and the most critical elements of teaching protocols.

REFERENCES

1. Christopher KL, Wood RP II, Eckert RC, et al. Vocal cord dysfunction presenting as asthma: a multi-disciplinary analysis of five patients. N Engl J Med 1983;308:1566–70.
2. Chiang T, Marcinow AM, deSilva BW, et al. Exercise-induced paradoxical vocal fold motion disorder: diagnosis and management. Laryngoscope 2013;123:727–31.
3. Earles J, Burton K, Kellar M. Psychophysiologic treatment of vocal cord dysfunction. Ann Allergy Asthma Immunol 2003;90:669–71.
4. Hodges H. Speech therapy for functional respiratory disorders. In: Anbar RD, editor. Functional respiratory Springer Science & Business Media. New York: Humana Press; 2012. p. 251–78.
5. Kayani S, Shannon DC. Vocal cord dysfunction associated with exercise in adolescent girls. Chest 1998;113:540–2.
6. Kuppersmith BA, Rosen DS, Wiatrak B. Functional stridor in adolescents. J Adolesc Health 1993;14:166–71.
7. Marcinow AM, Thompson J, Chiang T, et al. Paradoxical vocal fold motion disorder in the elite athlete: experience at a large division I university. Laryngoscope 2014;124:1425–30.
8. Marcinow AM, Thompson J, Forrest LA, et al. Irritant-induced paradoxical vocal fold motion disorder: diagnosis and management. Otolaryngol Head Neck Surg 2015;153(6):996–1000.
9. Martin RJ, Blager FB, Gay ML, et al. Paradoxic vocal cord motion in presumed asthmatics. Semin Respir Med 1987;8(4):332–7.
10. Mathers-Schmidt BA. Paradoxical vocal fold motion: a tutorial on a complex disorder and the speech-language pathologist's role. Am J Speech Lang Pathol 2001;10:111–25.
11. Mathers-Schmidt BA, Brilla LR. Inspiratory muscle training in exercise-induced paradoxical vocal fold motion. J Voice 2005;19(4):635–44.
12. Pinho SMR, Tsuji DH, Sennes L, et al. Paradoxical vocal fold movement: a case report. J Voice 1997;11(3):368–72.
13. Sandage MJ, Zelazny SK. Paradoxical vocal fold motion in children and adolescents. Lang Speech Hear Serv Sch 2004;35:353–62.

14. Sullivan MD, Heywood BM, Beukelman DR. A treatment for vocal cord dysfunction in female athletes: an outcome study. Laryngoscope 2001;111:1751–5.
15. Denipah N, Dominguez CM, Kraai EP, et al. Acute management of paradoxical vocal fold motion (vocal cord dysfunction). Ann Emerg Med 2017;1:18–23.
16. Hicks M, Brugman SM, Katial R. Vocal cord dysfunction/paradoxical vocal fold motion. Prim Care 2008;35:81–103.
17. Rundell KW, Weiss P. Exercise-induced bronchoconstriction and vocal cord dysfunction: two sides of the same coin? Curr Sports Med Rep 2013;12(1):41–6.
18. Patel NJ, Jorgenson C, Kuhn J, et al. Concurrent laryngeal abnormalities in patients with paradoxical vocal fold dysfunction. Otolaryngol Head Neck Surg 2004;130:686–9.
19. Morris MJ, Allan PF, Perkins PJ. Vocal cord dysfunction: etiologies and treatment. Clin Pulm Med 2006;13(2):73–86.
20. Altman KW, Mirza N, Ruiz C, et al. Paradoxical vocal fold motion: presentation and treatment options. J Voice 2000;14(1):99–103.
21. Goldman J, Muers M. Vocal cord dysfunction and wheezing. Thorax 1991;46:401–4.
22. Gallena SJK, Kerins MR. Nonspecific chronic cough and paradoxical vocal fold motion disorder in pediatric patients. Semin Speech Lang 2013;34:116–28.
23. Johnston KL, Bradford H, Hodges HL, et al. The Olin EILOBI breathing techniques: description and initial case series of novel respiratory retraining strategies for athletes with exercise-induced laryngeal obstruction. J Voice 2017. [Epub ahead of print].
24. Graham S, Deardorff EH, Johnston KL, et al. The fortuitous discovery of the Olin EILOBI breathing techniques: a case study. J Voice 2017. [Epub ahead of print].
25. De Guzman V, Ballif CL, Maurer R, et al. Validation of dyspnea index in adolescents with exercise-induced paradoxical vocal fold motion. JAMA 2014;140:823–8.
26. Maat RC, Hilland M, Røksund OD, et al. Exercise-induced laryngeal obstruction: natural history and effect of surgical treatment. Eur Arch Otorhinolaryngol 2011;268(10):1485–92.
27. Volianitis S, McConnell AK, Koutedakis Y, et al. Inspiratory muscle training improved rowing performance. Med Sci Sports Exerc 2001;33(5):803–9.
28. Baker SE, Sapienza CM, Martin D, et al. Inspiratory pressure threshold training for upper airway limitation: a case of bilateral abductor vocal fold paralysis. J Voice 2002;17:384–94.
29. Boutellier U. Respiratory muscle fitness and exercise endurance in healthy humans. Med Sci Sports Exerc 1998;30(7):1167–72.
30. Kellerman BA, Martin AD, Davenport PW. Inspiratory strengthening effects of resistive load detection and magnitude estimation. Med Sci Sports Exerc 2000;32(11):1859–67.
31. Koessler W, Wanke T, Winkler G, et al. 2 years' experience with inspiratory muscle training in patients with neuromuscular disorders. Chest 2001;120:765–9.
32. Sapienza CM, Brown J, Martin D, et al. Inspiratory pressure threshold training for glottal airway limitation in laryngeal papilloma. J Voice 1999;13:382–8.
33. Williams JS, Wongsathikun J, Boon SM, et al. Inspiratory muscle training fails to improve endurance capacity in athletes. Med Sci Sports Exerc 2002;34(7):1194–8.
34. Bastian RW, Magorsky MJ. Laryngeal image feedback. Laryngoscope 1987;97:1346–9.
35. Olin JT, Deardorff EH, Fan EM, et al. Therapeutic laryngoscopy during exercise: A novel non-surgical therapy for refractory EILO. Pediatr Pulmonol 2016. https://doi.org/10.1002/ppul.23634.

36. Reuben AD, Harris AR. Heliox for asthma in the emergency department: a review of the literature. Emerg Med J 2004;21:131–5.
37. Weir M. Vocal cord dysfunction mimics asthma and may respond to heliox. Clin Pediatr 2002;41(1):37–41.
38. Ulhoa CAG, Larner L. Helium-oxygen (heliox) mixture in airway obstruction. J Pediatr (Rio J) 2000;76(1):73–8.
39. Kim IK, Cocoran T. Recent developments in heliox therapy for asthma and bronchiolitis. Clin Pediatr Emerg Med 2009;10(2):68–74.
40. Hashemian SM, Fallahian F. The use of heliox in critical care. Int J Crit Illn Inj Sci 2014;4(2):138–42.
41. Reisner C, Borish L. Heliox therapy for acute vocal cord dysfunction. Chest 1995; 108(5):1477.

Exercise-Induced Laryngeal Obstruction and Performance Psychology
Using the Mind as a Diagnostic and
Therapeutic Target

J. Tod Olin, MD, MSCS[a],*, Erika Westhoff (Carlson), MA, CC-AASP[b]

KEYWORDS

- Exercise-induced laryngeal obstruction • Performance psychology • Therapy
- Vocal cord dysfunction • Paradoxical vocal fold motion

KEY POINTS

- Recent literature suggests that patients with exercise-induced laryngeal obstruction do not exhibit the mental health patterns described in seminal literature on inducible laryngeal obstruction, but rather are mentally healthy.
- With the performance psychologist or mental skills coach, it is reasonable to assess and restructure patient belief systems and thought patterns regarding the relationship between exercise and episodes of respiratory distress.
- Moving forward, there is adequate rationale to study the use of performance psychology as an adjunctive therapy for patients with exercise-induced laryngeal obstruction.

INTRODUCTION

Exercise-induced laryngeal obstruction (EILO), previously known as vocal cord dysfunction and paradoxic vocal fold motion, is a condition that causes severe shortness of breath during exercise in patients across a spectrum of athletic levels.[1,2] The mechanism of disease remains enigmatic, although several investigators have postulated a variety of contributing factors, including anatomic factors (airway size and pliability), upper airway reactivity, extrinsic factors (including postnasal drip and gastroesophageal reflux), and behavioral health factors (such as a stress-prone personality, perfectionistic tendencies, attributional style, and impaired self-efficacy).[3–9]

[a] Department of Pediatrics, National Jewish Health, 1400 Jackson Street, Box J-317, Denver, CO 80206, USA; [b] Erika Westhoff Performance, Pleasanton, CA, USA
* Corresponding author.
E-mail address: olint@njhealth.org

Immunol Allergy Clin N Am 38 (2018) 303–315
https://doi.org/10.1016/j.iac.2018.01.004   immunology.theclinics.com
0889-8561/18/© 2018 Elsevier Inc. All rights reserved.

Since the early reports of this condition, clinicians and researchers have documented an observation that behavioral health factors are associated with the pathogenesis of disease.[10] Later reports of cohorts strongly emphasized this possibility although with rare exception,[11,12] research in the 1990s and 2000s did not routinely stratify patients based on isolation of symptoms to exercise grouping of patients with EILO and inducible laryngeal obstruction (ILO), also known as vocal cord dysfunction, caused by a variety of triggers.[4,5,13,14] This lack of stratification may be important, because it is possible that the behavioral health features of patients with symptoms limited to exercise differ from those who experience symptoms in response to irritants or overt situational stresses.[15–18] At the current time, there is no published spectrum of psychiatric and psychological disease, personality disorders, or dysfunctional traits and coping mechanisms in patients with isolated EILO.

Despite the lack of prospective behavioral health assessments that are isolated to patients with EILO, this review aims to achieve a few specific goals. First, we summarize some of the literature that characterizes the behavioral health features of the prototypical patient with EILO, drawing comparisons with the general ILO patient. This discussion will include some of the chronic features of personality documented in the literature as well as descriptions of thoughts verbalized by patients struggling with symptoms. Second, we discuss some of the available assessment tools that can quantify some of the features noted. Finally, we discuss in detail some therapeutic approaches from the perspective of the performance psychology. We will use a few cases to demonstrate key concepts.

CASE 1

A 15-year-old female competitive swimmer presented with several months of exertional dyspnea in the context of asthma. Evaluation before specialty care included spirometry with mild obstruction and a positive response to bronchodilators, as well as a normal computed tomography scan of the sinuses. Therapeutic trials before specialty care included daily fluticasone 100 μg/salmeterol 50 μg, which was escalated to fluticasone 250 μg/salmeterol 50 μg as well as montelukast 10 mg/d, nasal steroids, and oral antihistamines. She was then evaluated by an allergist, who optimized nasal care (with nasal saline washes and improved in nasal steroid technique) and transitioned combination controller therapy to a metered dose inhaler formulation with spacer (of comparable dosage). She was later referred to our exertional dyspnea program for an incomplete response of exertional dyspnea to therapy, described by the patient as "a block near the top of my lungs." Symptoms only occurred during high-intensity swimming and were not clearly associated with audible stridor, although the patient noted that she was unable to assess her breathing while underwater. Initially, the dyspnea was quite frightening for the patient, although this response had improved somewhat. There was associated cough during and after exercise. There was no associated chest pain, pallor, cyanosis, presyncope, or syncope. Events generally occurred after 7 minutes of intense exercise and returned to baseline after about 10 minutes.

Physical examination was normal. Spirometry demonstrated mildly obstructed airflow (forced expiratory volume in 1 second [FEV_1]/forced vital capacity of 0.78) with an 8% improvement in FEV_1 in response to bronchodilator. Continuous laryngoscopy during exercise testing demonstrated excellent fitness (peak oxygen consumption of 51 mL/kg/min at our altitude of 1600 m above sea level), no desaturation, no postexertional bronchoconstriction (7% increase), and mild inspiratory glottic adduction associated with a faint audible stridor and inspiratory blunting of exercise flow volume loops.

Based on the constellation of findings, she was diagnosed with EILO in addition to her asthma and referred to a speech-language pathologist. Given an incomplete response to therapy to basic respiratory retraining, she performed 2 sessions of therapeutic laryngoscopy during exercise, which greatly improved her symptoms over a few weeks. However, several weeks after this improvement, the patient, the patient's mother, and the patient's swimming coach all noted a trend in which the patient seemed to struggle mainly during high-stakes competitions, remaining relatively symptom free during training and other competitions. For this reason, she was referred to a mental skills coach.

CASE 2

A 17-year-old male competitive swimmer was referred to our exertional dyspnea program for clinical suspicion of EILO despite a negative preexercise and postexercise laryngoscopy. He described the symptom of interest as a complete inability to inhale, primarily during races, but did not note audible stridor. Symptoms often occurred in less than 1 minute and almost immediately resolved upon exercise cessation. Previous asthma therapy was ineffective in terms of the symptom of interest.

The patient's physical examination was normal. Spirometry demonstrated mildly obstructed airflow (FEV_1/forced vital capacity of 0.74) with FEV_1 improvement of 8% with albuterol. A methacholine challenge was negative. Continuous laryngoscopy during exercise demonstrated normal fitness (peak oxygen consumption of 42 mL/kg/min), no desaturation or airflow decrease after exercise, and mild inspiratory glottic adduction with moderate inspiratory arytenoid prolapse and inspiratory blunting of exercise flow volume loops at peak work capacity. In addition to respiratory retraining directed by a speech-language pathologist, the patient performed 2 sessions of therapeutic laryngoscopy during exercise.

This patient also initially improved, but later struggled in a high-stakes competition. During a 100-m butterfly race, the patient experienced dyspnea so profound that he stopped swimming after roughly 60 m (roughly 30 seconds). The results of this event were highly discouraging and carried over to a later inability to complete entire practices. After discussions of pre-race anxiety, the patient was referred to a mental skills coach.

BEHAVIORAL HEALTH DOMAINS AND EXERCISE-INDUCED LARYNGEAL OBSTRUCTION

Examining the interactions between behavioral health and EILO, and recognizing that the identification of potential problems may lead to differential therapeutic approaches across domain, we consider different domains of behavioral health. Specifically, we briefly reflect on the literature devoted to psychopathology (defined as the study of mental disorders), personality types (defined as a group of personality traits that exist together), and belief systems and attributional styles (defined as the manner in which people explain experiences) that may affect the response to stress.

MENTAL HEALTH CONCERNS: DID EARLY LITERATURE MISREPRESENT PATIENTS WITH EXERCISE-INDUCED LARYNGEAL OBSTRUCTION?

A number of mental health disorders have been associated with ILO and this association may be somewhat misleading when considering patients with isolated EILO. Early descriptions of ILO conveyed the impression of a strong perceived link between the condition and psychopathology, as evidenced by names for the condition including Munchausen's stridor, psychogenic stridor, and factitious asthma.[19–21]

The first retrospective reviews of a large cohort supported this initial impression; Newman and colleagues[17] reported a very high prevalence of mental health diagnoses in an unstratified ILO cohort.

More systematic approaches emerged in the decades that followed. In 2008, in a series of 30 patients with unspecified ILO, roughly one-half of the study population were noted via the Hospital Anxiety and Depression scale to demonstrate abnormally high levels of anxiety.[5] Another cohort of unstratified ILO patients with a notable age skew toward patients in their 50s and 60s, assessed with the Minnesota Multiphasic Personality Inventory-2, demonstrated elevated scores on the hypochondriasis scale, mildly elevated on the depression scale, highly elevated on the hysteria scale, without elevation on the anxiety scale, demonstrating a pattern referred to as the "conversion V" profile.[13]

In contrast, case series and case reports of patients with symptoms isolated to exercise paint a different picture than the initial description of patients struggling with factitious stridor, conversion disorder, sexual abuse, and hypochondriasis. To this day, although large series are not available, characteristic patients described in the literature are noted to be anxious.[22] However, Lakin and associates,[1] in what may have been the first description of EILO, acknowledged a contrast between the index patient and those patients with symptoms described outside of exercise previously. Later, a series of adolescent patients with symptoms largely localized to exercise was described in which 55% acknowledged "important social stresses," although the authors do not note the type or degree of psychological symptomatology present in general ILO reports.[23] Some other series have also reported decreased frequencies of psychiatric illness in athletic populations, without quantifying the frequencies of specific disorders.[11,12] In a recent review, authors describe a clinical perception that the majority of patients with EILO do not exhibit psychopathology, but rather an appropriate behavioral response to severe respiratory distress.[24]

Given the stigma associated with some of the mental health conditions associated with general ILO, including malingering, conversion disorder, and a history of sexual abuse, there is value in clearly distinguishing patients with symptoms of isolated EILO as potential behavioral health assessments and therapies could vastly differ across the 2 populations.[14,16,25–27]

PERSONALITY TYPES

Independent of mental health disorders, it is possible that personality features have a relation to the presence or absence of EILO symptoms or the severity of symptoms when present. True personality disorders are different than other mental health diagnoses in that they represent entrenched behavior patterns, defined during childhood and the adolescent years, that are somewhat less responsive to intervention than other mental health diagnoses.

Multiple authors have noticed personality features that stand out in prototypical patients with EILO, including the type A or hurried (high-stress) personality.[28] In one of the initial series devoted to adolescent patients with EILO, Landwehr and colleagues[3] discussed a notable trend of patients demonstrating excellent academic performance, despite the fact that the case series was devoted to exercise-induced symptoms, an observation atypical for case series descriptions of most diseases. Common characteristics of patients with type A personalities include time urgency, multitasking, ultracompetitiveness, rapid speech patterns, manipulative control, hyperaggressiveness, and free-floating hostility. There may be relevance in this observation given the long, documented relationship between behavior traits of the type A personality and the stress response.

In our local experience, another prominent stress-prone personality feature often seen in the EILO athlete population is perfectionism. The prototypical perfectionist strives to avoid failure and please those close to them by imposing unreasonably challenging self-standards.

There has never been a spectrum of personality traits and types published specifically in a population of patients with EILO. However, work in the area may provide therapeutic benefit in terms of identifying modifiable features within patients that have an effect on breathing. It is possible that the true disease mechanism may be related, causally or in association. It is possible that the identification of personality features could help to identify EILO from a diagnostic perspective. It is also possible that treatment could target specific personality features with the global goal of affecting EILO symptoms or that treatment or communication styles could be stratified based on personality features.

BELIEFS, ATTRIBUTIONAL STYLES, AND THE RESPONSE TO STRESS

Beliefs, independent of true psychopathology or personality traits, are important drivers of behavior, and may have relevance to a patient's ability to deal with the situational stress that is present during EILO.[24] Especially for otherwise mentally healthy athletes, it may be important to examine how existing beliefs may be shaping coping behavior before and during stressful events. There are a few specific models for thinking about these concepts for all individuals, including athletes.

Clinically, we have noticed multiple instances of disruptive thinking. One type of sentiment that is commonly expressed is a decreased willingness to participate in sport or high-intensity exercise owing to EILO, which is perceived by the patient to be a permanent, unchanging entity. A second type of sentiment that is commonly expressed at our center relates to a belief that EILO is not, and cannot be, independently controllable by a patient.

These specific sentiments are specifically addressed by prominent theoretic work in the field of performance psychology. In 1 model of belief systems relevant to performance psychology, now known as the social cognitive model of achievement motivation, there is a clear distinction drawn between incremental beliefs (which are viewed as malleable or controllable) and entity beliefs (which are viewed as fixed). This model is the theoretic foundation of the growth and fixed mindsets, and is based in the theory that core cognitive processing and situational appraisals lead to the anxiety response.[29–31] In the context of EILO, a theoretic example of an entity belief is thought such as, "EILO is stopping me from playing, I can't do it." The theoretic example of an incremental belief is, "I have allowed EILO to take over, and can take control back." It is possible that these hypothetical beliefs could be shaped by factors such as delayed time to diagnosis or poor response to the initial asthma or EILO therapy, features that have been noted in the literature for decades.[17] Entity beliefs have been linked to maladaptive cognitive, behavioral, and affective outcomes, such as decreased motivation and withdrawal from tasks. Conversely, incremental beliefs are associated with more positive outcomes, such as greater motivation and task persistence, and lower anxiety.[32,33]

A second explanatory model deals with the concept of self-efficacy, defined as the set of beliefs in one's capabilities to organize and execute courses of action required to generate desired results.[34] Work in self-efficacy was foundational to linking self-beliefs with behavioral responses. It is possible that patients with robust perceptions of self-efficacy are more resilient to stress, which may have relevance to EILO occurrences and treatment.

There is no specific literature relating these relatively new psychological constructs and EILO, although the assessment and manipulation of these areas may prove fruitful from a diagnostic and therapeutic perspective going forward. A need exists to investigate this area in terms of relevance to future therapeutic approaches.

RELATING COGNITIVE–BEHAVIORAL PHENOMENA TO DISEASE MECHANISM

At the current time, it is very challenging to mechanistically relate cognitive–behavioral observations in a variety of domains in patients with EILO to a final common anatomic pathway of upper airway obstruction that occurs during high-intensity exercise. Clearly, some of the pathologic states, personality traits, and belief systems are associated with increased levels of anxiety and perceived situational stress. In accordance with this assumption that increased anxiety and stress levels are present in prototype patients, and observations that these scenarios have been associated with increased sympathetic activity, it is reasonable to hypothesize that a dysregulated sympathetic response could predispose patients with EILO to events.[35] Complicating the study of this area is the cyclical nature of the relationship between respiratory distress, anxiety, and stress responses. Debate remains regarding whether symptoms are a result of behavioral makeup and responses, or if EILO shapes the responses. Clearly, there are a variety of opinions related to causation between these entities.[24]

ASSESSING BEHAVIORAL MAKEUP AND BELIEFS

The performance psychology assessment of patients with EILO is not standardized across centers nor have anecdotal reports or guidelines been published. Based on the domains of anxiety-based or depressive psychopathology, maladaptive personality traits, and disruptive belief systems and attributional styles, we propose considering the following assessments in conjunction with consultation with performance psychology specialists in select patients. Underscoring any recommendations related to assessment is the concept that metrics should only be used by providers that have knowledge of the specific test properties of the metric.

ASSESSMENT OF DEPRESSION AND ANXIETY

The assessment of depression and anxiety is possible via a number of metrics that have been validated in general populations. The Depression Anxiety Stress Scale 21 is one patient-centered outcome that has been validated and is easy to administrate.[36] This metric is considered useful because it may identify individuals who fall short of a clinical diagnosis of anxiety, but who present with a high risk of further problems such as moderate, situational stress.[36] Another metric, the Hospital Anxiety and Depression Scale, has been used in the context of patients with ILO.[5] Advantages of this metric include its ability to assess the existence and symptom severity of anxiety disorders and depression in a variety of populations.[37]

PERSONALITY ASSESSMENT

A number of metrics that quantify domains of personality type exist as well and are available commercially. The assessment of personality has not been related to treatment outcomes in EILO. We hypothesize that an understanding of patient personality may be helpful in the future for diagnostic reasons (in terms of identifying patients with personality traits that predict a response to therapy) and therapeutic reasons (in terms of identifying patients with needs for specific communication strategies). Further research is needed to identify personality metrics that could benefit care of patients with EILO.

BELIEF SYSTEMS ASSESSMENT

The assessment of belief systems has also not been tied to treatment outcomes in EILO. We hypothesize that a few basic assessments are important based only on our clinical experience. First, it is important to assess the level of patient understanding regarding the physiologic nature of their EILO diagnosis as well as the degree of patient acceptance of the diagnosis. Additionally, we attempt to assess patient perception of the degree of symptom permanence that exists, as well as the degree of perceived control over symptoms, understanding that perceived consequences of symptoms and thoughts may be linked to perceptions of control over symptoms.[38] Finally, there may be value in exploring the degree of motivation that exists within a patient. This can include motivations to continue with sport as well as motivation to participate in respiratory retraining and performance psychology intervention.

PERFORMANCE PSYCHOLOGY INTERVENTION AS A THERAPY FOR EXERCISE-INDUCED LARYNGEAL OBSTRUCTION

There are no guidelines or published studies of performance psychology interventions for patients with EILO. The specific place within the spectrum of treatments has yet to be established. Nonetheless, multiple reviews have concluded that potential therapeutic benefit to psychology intervention in EILO may exist.[39,40] We present an approach overview that could be considered by performance psychologists, working as part of a multidisciplinary team engaging patients with EILO as a primary complaint (**Box 1**). We strongly endorse the medical treatment of behavioral health diagnoses that are amenable to treatment, including major depressive disorder and generalized anxiety disorder. This is consistent with reports back to the initial descriptions of ILO and EILO.[15,41] This review will not discuss specific approaches to address specific personality types. This section focuses on modifying stress and beliefs as a therapeutic intervention.

GOAL SETTING

Within the field of performance psychology, it is fairly common to initially devote therapeutic time to goal setting, that is, focusing on both measures of performance and measures of process improvement. Goal setting can include patient-derived metrics of breathing improvement in the context of sport performance and stress responses.

Box 1
Proposed framework for performance psychology interventions in exercise-induced laryngeal obstruction

Goal setting

Baseline relaxation

Visualization

Cognitive restructuring
  Journaling
  Reframing

Examples of such thinking could include patient self-assessment of thought patterns before competition and during respiratory distress as well as self-assessment of respiratory responses to characteristic stress experienced during training and competition.

BASELINE STRESS REDUCTION

Patients may benefit from the acquisition of teachable skills, designed to lower baseline levels of stress. Diaphragmatic breathing is a simple technique that reduces sympathetic drive.[42] Although challenging to perform during high-intensity exercise, is important to note that this technique may be most beneficial at rest. It may be used as a precursor to progressive relaxation, defined as a technique that relies on repeatedly contracting and relaxing local and regional muscle groups, which also may contribute to physiologic stress reduction.[43]

VISUALIZATION AND THE USE OF IMAGERY

Visualization, or mental rehearsal, is an approach that may restructure thoughts that occur acutely and chronically. In this technique, patients can imagine imagery, relating to all senses, of commonly encountered situations. The technique, when focused on specifically troublesome situations, may desensitize patients to stressful stimuli, allowing the body to manage stress more effectively. Patients can visualize somewhat longer periods of time that are characterized by success with respect to EILO symptoms. Patients can also, in a time of rest, visualize specific respiratory maneuvers or thoughts that they choose to use therapeutically to build coordination and execution skills. Patients with EILO, thus, can use imagery to both theoretically prevent an episode and to rehearse skills to help them recover from an episode of respiratory distress. Evidence for the use of visualization and sport dates back to the 1980s, when motor skill rehearsal with imagery was shown to reinforce the neural tracts responsible for motor performance, leading to improved coordination results.[44] Subsequent studies supported these findings and showed that imagery routines full of details about specific skills and patterns were especially beneficial.[45–47]

COGNITIVE RESTRUCTURING

There are also approaches to restructuring belief systems and thought patterns.[48] Cognitive restructuring, defined as a coping technique in which patients are guided to substitute negative, self-defeating thoughts with positive, affirming thoughts has been found to be effective as a stress reduction strategy.[49–51] In this approach, patients change perceptions of stressors from threatening to nonthreatening. This experience can be extrapolated to the treatment of EILO.

One approach to restructuring thoughts includes rationally analyzing situations that have caused specific problems with respect to EILO and specific thoughts that could be classified as negative self-talk. Journaling about these situations and thoughts is a technique that patients can use to gain insight with goals of modifying situations and ultimately restructuring thoughts into more facilitative beliefs. It is fairly straightforward for patients to reflect on experiences with EILO symptoms and situational variables associated with symptoms. These reflections may include factors that are outside of the control of patients (ambient temperature, competitive opposition) and factors that are under the control of patients (hydration status, precompetition routine). With proper reflection, patients also can write about whether or not thoughts represent past observations or predictions of the future. Similarly, patients can self-assess the degree of rationality behind a thought, the degree of permanence that is associated with that thought, and the relationship between a thought and reality when viewed from a distance. It is felt that journaling may provide awareness into factors that may be better managed before exercise and provide a therapeutic degree of distance between a specific patient and a specific thought.[52]

Another approach relates to reframing thoughts is related to perceptions of stress. Evidence suggests that there is variability in the perception of the significance of symptoms related situational stress (with some athletes viewing these symptoms as facilitative and others viewing the symptoms as debilitative) and variability in the ability to cope independently with the symptoms, despite the fact that physical description of the symptoms is comparable across groups.[45] Although individuals who view symptoms as facilitative tend to also be individuals with adaptive coping mechanisms, individuals who perceive symptoms as debilitative often do not have the mental skills set necessary to independently reframe these symptoms as positive.[53–55] This finding might suggest that specific individuals could notably be targeted and benefit from external intervention via a performance psychologist to improve adaptive mental skills, including reframing.[53]

In the specific population of patients with EILO, none of these interventions has been tested. There are very notable barriers to study, including the assessment of intervention delivery and the assessment of patient outcomes. However, given the long history of association between behavioral health phenomena and EILO symptoms and impact, there is adequate rationale to study these and other behavioral health interventions in populations with EILO.

CASE RESOLUTIONS AND REFLECTIONS

The patients described in cases 1 and 2 demonstrated several important concepts at the interface of EILO and performance psychology. First, the patients presented without overt psychopathology. Next, there were initial challenges in terms of establishing acceptance of the diagnosis, despite the incomplete response of symptoms to aggressive asthma therapy, because many of the clinical and physiologic findings were not clearly indicative of EILO, including the patients' inability to detect stridor, the time course of symptoms (in case 1), and mild inspiratory glottic adduction on continuous laryngoscopy during exercise. Finally, although most symptoms resolved in response to behavioral interventions, symptoms isolated to high-stakes competitions persisted.

From a behavioral health and mental skills perspective, patient 1 did not carry formal mental health diagnoses. She was a conscientious student and a very motivated athlete with goals to be a top-ranked swimmer in her state and earn a college scholarship. At baseline, she was extremely frustrated by her breathing symptoms. Before competitions, she struggled with low confidence and notable anxiety, citing her concern for impending EILO symptoms as the source of these feelings. Patient 1 completed a 6-week program to learn, practice, and systematically apply fundamental mental skills, including goal setting, cognitive restructuring, imagery, emotion control strategies, journaling, and accountability tracking (defined as the setting and tracking of preparation goals). The program was designed to help her manage stress-inducing thoughts, behaviors, and emotions before and during strenuous workouts and races. Patient 1 then continued on to an additional 6-week program to fine-tune her skills with coaching support and to practice the skills in a variety of competitive situations ranging from typical team workouts to state-level competition. Patient 1 was highly compliant with her mental skills program, completing nearly 100% of her assigned tasks throughout the program, and was able to gain a strong sense of confidence and control over her preparation and performance. As her control and confidence grew, EILO symptoms subsided and she was able to consistently perform in practice and competitions to her full potential with no respiratory disruption.

Patient 2 was a diligent high school senior student without a formal mental health diagnosis who had aspirations to win team and individual state championships in swimming. At the time of his presentation for mental skills training, EILO symptoms often prevented completion of practice. At baseline, he was highly frustrated with and discouraged by EILO symptoms, leading to an acknowledgment of a lack of hope for improvement. Before competitions, the patient acknowledged notable anxiety in general, as well as specific concern about EILO episodes. He initially expressed skepticism in the usefulness of mental skills training given an unfruitful prior experience with another provider unfamiliar with EILO. He overcame his skepticism and committed to a 10-week program that was structurally similar in terms of focus and content to the program used by patient 1. Patient 2 was able to find success within a few weeks of applying the mental skills before preseason training sessions and during high-intensity sets. The patient incrementally increased work intensity while maintaining a focus on mental skills as his season started, and noted that he was unable to induce EILO symptoms during training. This progress gave him the confidence to start his season and a sense of control over his symptoms. With use of preworkout, pre-race, and in-race routines, he acknowledged control over his thoughts, behaviors, and emotions in those respective situations. He remained symptom free throughout the season, won a state championship with his team and an individual state championship in the 100-yard backstroke, and committed to swim in college.

These cases demonstrate an observation that patients with EILO can be mentally healthy and yet struggle notably in high-stakes sporting competitions that are increasingly common in some cultures worldwide. Especially for adolescents, it is reasonable to hypothesize that some patients may not have developed the skills to calmly approach competitions, the results of which are linked to important consequences such as college scholarships. Consistent with hypotheses that stress is a factor in EILO and those with stress-prone personality traits may be predisposed to EILO, today's youth sport culture may contribute to the incidence of EILO. In this line of thinking, EILO outcomes for selected individuals may notably improve as a result of partnerships with performance psychologists or mental skills coaches who help these patients to effectively cope with stress they encounter during competition.

SUMMARY

EILO has long been characterized as a condition that is often seen in patients with anxiety-spectrum mental health concerns, type A personality types, and perfectionistic thought patterns. These observations have not been characterized at the level of large populations and the mechanistic significance of these observations is unclear. Several metrics exist for the assessment mental health and personality traits. Negative thought patterns can be assessed through conversational techniques. Moving forward, there is reasonable theoretic and case-based rationale to study performance psychology interventions as a therapeutic modality for EILO.

REFERENCES

1. Lakin RC, Metzger WJ, Haughey BH. Upper airway obstruction presenting as exercise-induced asthma. Chest 1984;86(3):499–501.

2. Christensen PM, Heimdal JH, Christopher KL, et al. ERS/ELS/ACCP 2013 international consensus conference nomenclature on inducible laryngeal obstructions. Eur Respir Rev 2015;24(137):445–50.
3. Landwehr LP, Wood RP, Blager FB, et al. Vocal cord dysfunction mimicking exercise-induced bronchospasm in adolescents. Pediatrics 1996;98(5):971–4.
4. Gavin LA, Wamboldt M, Brugman S, et al. Psychological and family characteristics of adolescents with vocal cord dysfunction. J Asthma 1998;35(5):409–17.
5. Dietrich M, Verdolini Abbott K, Gartner-Schmidt J, et al. The frequency of perceived stress, anxiety, and depression in patients with common pathologies affecting voice. J Voice 2008;22(4):472–88.
6. Mandell DL, Arjmand EM. Laryngomalacia induced by exercise in a pediatric patient. Int J Pediatr Otorhinolaryngol 2003;67(9):999–1003.
7. Tilles SA, Ayars AG, Picciano JF, et al. Exercise-induced vocal cord dysfunction and exercise-induced laryngomalacia in children and adolescents: the same clinical syndrome? Ann Allergy Asthma Immunol 2013;111(5):342–6.e1.
8. Morrison M, Rammage L, Emami AJ. The irritable larynx syndrome. J Voice 1999; 13(3):447–55.
9. Bucca C, Rolla G, Scappaticci E, et al. Extrathoracic and intrathoracic airway responsiveness in sinusitis. J Allergy Clin Immunol 1995;95(1 Pt 1):52–9.
10. McFadden ER Jr, Zawadski DK. Vocal cord dysfunction masquerading as exercise-induced asthma. a physiologic cause for "choking" during athletic activities. Am J Respir Crit Care Med 1996;153(3):942–7.
11. Chiang T, Marcinow AM, deSilva BW, et al. Exercise-induced paradoxical vocal fold motion disorder: diagnosis and management. Laryngoscope 2013;123(3): 727–31.
12. Marcinow AM, Thompson J, Chiang T, et al. Paradoxical vocal fold motion disorder in the elite athlete: experience at a large division I university. Laryngoscope 2014;124(6):1425–30.
13. Husein OF, Husein TN, Gardner R, et al. Formal psychological testing in patients with paradoxical vocal fold dysfunction. Laryngoscope 2008;118(4):740–7.
14. Forrest LA, Husein T, Husein O. Paradoxical vocal cord motion: classification and treatment. Laryngoscope 2012;122(4):844–53.
15. Christopher KL, Wood RP, Eckert RC, et al. Vocal-cord dysfunction presenting as asthma. N Engl J Med 1983;308(26):1566–70.
16. Freedman MR, Rosenberg SJ, Schmaling KB. Childhood sexual abuse in patients with paradoxical vocal cord dysfunction. J Nerv Ment Dis 1991;179(5):295–8.
17. Newman KB, Mason UG III, Schmaling KB. Clinical features of vocal cord dysfunction. Am J Respir Crit Care Med 1995;152(4 Pt 1):1382–6.
18. Balasubramaniam SK, O'Connell EJ, Sachs MI, et al. Recurrent exercise-induced stridor in an adolescent. Ann Allergy 1986;57(4):243, 287–8.
19. Patterson R, Schatz M, Horton M. Munchausen's stridor: non-organic laryngeal obstruction. Clin Allergy 1974;4(3):307–10.
20. Lacy TJ, McManis SE. Psychogenic stridor. Gen Hosp Psychiatry 1994;16(3): 213–23.
21. Downing ET, Braman SS, Fox MJ, et al. Factitious asthma. Physiological approach to diagnosis. JAMA 1982;248(21):2878–81.
22. Palla J, Friedman AD. Paradoxical vocal cord motion in pediatric patients. Pediatr Ann 2016;45(5):e184–188.
23. Powell DM, Karanfilov BI, Beechler KB, et al. Paradoxical vocal cord dysfunction in juveniles. Arch Otolaryngol Head Neck Surg 2000;126(1):29–34.

24. Roksund OD, Heimdal JH, Clemm H, et al. Exercise inducible laryngeal obstruction: diagnostics and management. Paediatr Respir Rev 2017;21:86–94.
25. Geist R, Tallett SE. Diagnosis and management of psychogenic stridor caused by a conversion disorder. Pediatrics 1990;86(2):315–7.
26. Smith MS. Acute psychogenic stridor in an adolescent athlete treated with hypnosis. Pediatrics 1983;72(2):247–8.
27. Meltzer EO, Orgel HA, Kemp JP, et al. Vocal cord dysfunction in a child with asthma. J Asthma 1991;28(2):141–5.
28. Brugman SM, Simons SM. Vocal cord dysfunction: don't mistake it for asthma. Phys Sportsmed 1998;26(5):63–74.
29. Gardner L, Vella S, Magee C. The relationship between implicit beliefs, anxiety, and attributional style and high-level soccer players. J Appl Sport Psychol 2015;27(4):398–411.
30. Dweck C, Leggett E. The social-cognitive approach to motivation and personality. Psychol Rev 1988;95(2):256–73.
31. Lazarus R. How emotions influence performance in competitive sports. Sport Psychol 2000;14(3):229–52.
32. Dweck C, Chiu CY, Hong Y. Implicit theories in their role in judgments and reactions: a world from two perspectives. Psychol Inq 1995;6(4):267–85.
33. Tamir M, John O, Srivastava S, et al. Implicit theories of emotion: effective and social outcomes across a major life transition. J Pers Soc Psychol 2007;95(4):731–44.
34. Bandura A. Self-efficacy mechanism in human agency. Am Psychol 1982;37(2):122–47.
35. Rice PL. Stress and health. 3rd edition. Wadsworth. Belmont (CA): Brooks/Cole Publishing Company; 1998.
36. Oei T, Sawang S, Goh Y, et al. Using the depression anxiety stress scale 21 (DASS-21) across cultures. Int J Psychol 2013;48(6):1018–29.
37. Bjelland I, Dahl AA, Haug TT, et al. The validity of the Hospital Anxiety and Depression Scale. An updated literature review. J Psychosom Res 2002;52(2):69–77.
38. Jones G, Swain A. Predispositions to experience debilitative and facilitative anxiety in elite and nonelite performers. Sport Psychol 1995;9(2):201–11.
39. Olin JT, Clary MS, Deardorff EH, et al. Inducible laryngeal obstruction during exercise: moving beyond vocal cords with new insights. Phys Sportsmed 2015;43(1):13–21.
40. Wilson JJ, Theis SM, Wilson EM. Evaluation and management of vocal cord dysfunction in the athlete. Curr Sports Med Rep 2009;8(2):65–70.
41. Kivity S, Bibi H, Schwarz Y, et al. Variable vocal cord dysfunction presenting as wheezing and exercise-induced asthma. J Asthma 1986;23(5):241–4.
42. Cahalin LP, Braga M, Matsuo Y, et al. Efficacy of diaphragmatic breathing in persons with chronic obstructive pulmonary disease: a review of the literature. J Cardiopulm Rehabil 2002;22(1):7–21.
43. Jacobson E. Modern treatment of tense patients. Springfield (IL): Thomas; 1970.
44. Harris D, Robinson W. The effects of skill level on EMG activity during internal and external imagery. J Sport Psychol 1986;8(2):105–11.
45. Tomas O, Hanton S. Anxiety responses and psychological skill use during the time leading up to a competition: theory and practice I. J Appl Sport Psychol 2007;19:379–97.
46. Paivio A. Cognitive and motivational functions of imagery in human performance. Can J Appl Sport Sci 1985;10(4):22S–8S.

47. Hall C. Imagery in sport and exercise. In: Handbook of sport psychology, vol. 2. 2001. p. 529–49.
48. Allen RJ. Human stress: its nature and control. Macmillan. Minneapolis (MN): Burgess Press; 1983.
49. Meichenbaum DH. A self-instructional approach to stress management: a proposal for stress inoculation. In: Spielberger CD, Sarason IG, editors. Stress and anxiety, vol. 2. New York: John Wiley & Sons; 1975.
50. Beck AT. Cognitive therapy and the emotional disorders. New York: International Universities Press; 1987.
51. Bandura A. Self-efficacy: the exercise of control. Freeman WH. New York: Worth Publishers; 1977.
52. Pennebaker JW, Colder M, Sharp LK. Accelerating the coping process. J Pers Soc Psychol 1990;58(3):528–37.
53. Hanton S, Connaughton D. Perceived control of anxiety and its relationship to self-confidence and performance. Res Q Exerc Sport 2002;73(1):87–97.
54. Hanton S, Mellalieu SD, Young SG. A qualitative investigation of the temporal patterning of the precompetitive anxiety response. J Sports Sci 2002;20(11): 911–28.
55. Hanton S, Jones G. The acquisition and development of cognitive skills and strategies: I. Making the butterflies fly in formation. Sport Psychol 1999;13(1):1–21.

Surgical Intervention for Exercise-Induced Laryngeal Obstruction

John-Helge Heimdal, MD, PhD[a,b,]*, Robert Maat, MD, PhD[c],
Leif Nordang, MD, PhD[d]

KEYWORDS

- Exercise • Laryngeal obstruction • Surgery • Laryngoplasty • Laryngomalacia

KEY POINTS

- The larynx quickly adapts to increased airflow during activity by inspiratory abduction of the aryepiglottic folds and vocal folds, which increases laryngeal aperture and decreases airflow resistance.
- Respiratory distress during strenuous exercise may be due to malfunction of this adaptive mechanism causing airflow obstruction in the larynx in patients with exercise-induced laryngeal obstruction (EILO).
- Laryngeal obstruction caused by inward rotation of aryepiglottic folds (supraglottic) shows similar findings as laryngomalacia in infants.
- Supraglottic laryngeal obstruction can be treated successfully with operative techniques that are also used in infants with laryngomalacia.
- Key elements in surgical treatment of EILO are presented including selection criteria for surgery, procedural details, outcomes, and risk factors.

 Video content accompanies this article at http://www.immunology.theclinics. com.

INTRODUCTION

During exercise, ventilation increases substantially. High airflow presumably causes notable negative pressures at narrow portions of the airways, including the larynx.

Disclosure Statement: The institution Haukeland University Hospital owns part of US patent # 11/134551, protecting the commercial rights of the CLE test.
[a] Department of Surgery, Haukeland University Hospital, Bergen University, Bergen, Norway; [b] Department of Otorhinolaryngology, Head and Neck Surgery, Haukeland University Hospital, Bergen University, Bergen, Norway; [c] Department of Otolaryngology, Röpcke-Zweers Hospital, Jan Weitkamplaan 4A, Hardenberg 7772 SE, The Netherlands; [d] Department of Surgical Sciences, Otorhinolaryngology, and Head and Neck Surgery, Uppsala University, Akademiska sjukhuset ing 78-79, Uppsala 75185, Sweden
* Corresponding author. Kirurgisk klinikk, Helse Bergen, Haukelandsveien 22, Bergen 5021, Norway.
E-mail address: john.heimdal@helse-bergen.no

Immunol Allergy Clin N Am 38 (2018) 317–324
https://doi.org/10.1016/j.iac.2018.01.005
0889-8561/18/© 2018 Elsevier Inc. All rights reserved.

immunology.theclinics.com

The larynx quickly adapts to the ventilatory demands of exercise through abduction of the glottic as well as supraglottic structures. Exercise-induced laryngeal obstruction (EILO) is a condition in which the larynx fails to remain fully patent during exercise because of dysfunction at a glottic or supraglottic level, and is characterized by typical symptoms of respiratory distress, dyspnea, stridor, and wheezing.[1]

Smith and colleagues described the condition in which EILO appeared largely isolated to the supraglottic structures. At the time of publication, the authors named their finding exercise-induced laryngomalacia (now known as EILO-supraglottic type), because they observed exertional laryngeal motions that appeared similar to those seen in infants with congenital laryngomalacia (CLM).[2,3] CLM, which is anatomically characterized by supraglottic laryngeal collapse, is the most common cause of stridor in infants and children, and similar conditions can occur throughout later childhood and adulthood.[4-6] Following initial reports of the condition, larger series were published, indicating that EILO-supraglottic type may be more common than previously recognized.[7] Patients with CLM that persists into childhood and adulthood may experience symptoms at rest[8,9] or during exercise alone.[5] There are reports indicating that CLM may increase the risk for EILO later in life, although a definite relationship between CLM and EILO has not yet been verified.[10]

Experience from the surgical treatment of CLM in infants has now been applied with clinical success in both children and youths with laryngomalacia, including some with EILO-supraglottic type.[2] Initial published case reports have been followed by larger series of patients treated surgically for EILO-supraglottic type.[11-13]

This article summarizes the surgical experience of the treatment of EILO-supraglottic type. It will describe the proposed indications for surgery, technical surgical considerations, outcomes, and complications. In areas not clearly guided by literature, surgical experience of the authors will be included.

LITERATURE REVIEW

Systematic searches in Medline databases, available through PubMed, have revealed descriptions of surgical treatment to a total of 64 EILO patients through the end of 2016 (**Table 1**). In recent years, the number of reports of successful treatment of supraglottic laryngeal collapse has increased substantially. Children and adults are included in these reports.

Table 1
Previous reports of surgically treated exercise-induced laryngeal obstruction

Authors, Year	Number	Examination
Smith et al,[2] 1995	1	Exercise and laryngoscopy
Bent et al,[14] 1996	2	Exercise and laryngoscopy
Björnsdóttir et al,[15] 2000	2	Exercise and laryngoscopy
Chemery et al,[20] 2002	1	Exercise simultaneous laryngoscopy
Mandell et al,[16] 2003	1	Laryngoscopy and spirometry
Richter et al,[6] 2008	3	Exercise laryngoscopy
Maat et al,[7] 2011	23	Exercise simultaneous laryngoscopy
Norlander et al,[12] 2015	14	Exercise simultaneous laryngoscopy
Mehlum et al,[13] 2016	17	Exercise simultaneous laryngoscopy
Total number	64	

Initial Case Reports

Smith and colleagues published the first paper describing supraglottoplasty in a patient with EILO-supraglottic type in 1995. Removal of the corniculate cartilages by laser resulted in improvement in aerobic endurance as measured by unspecified parameters in physical fitness testing.[2] Bent and colleagues[14] published a combined report that included the patient in the Smith report, as well as a second patient, and concluded a positive outcome in response to carbon dioxide laser supraglottoplasty featuring removal of the corniculate cartilages, as this second patient was significantly improved. In 2000, Björnsdóttir and colleagues described treatment with surgical removal of superfluous mucosa at the rim of the aryepiglottic folds and superfluous mucosa on the tuberculum corniculatum and tuberculum cuneiforme in 2 patients with EILO-supraglottic type.[15] A positive outcome was concluded based on unspecified resolution of symptoms that persisted for 3 years. In 2003, Mandell and Arjmand presented a case of surgical treatment of EILO-supraglottic type in a 10-year-old patient via staged sequential unilateral procedures featuring a releasing incision in each of the aryepiglottic folds and excision of the corniculate cartilages with surgical scissors.[16] A positive response was concluded based on a change in the inspiratory portion of the resting flow-volume loops and self-reported "increased exercise tolerance." Gessler and co-workers described a 27 year-old female with a condition that they described as an adult type of laryngomalacia characterized by inspiratory stridor.[8] This specific patient described symptom onset during exercise followed by symptom persistence for days at rest (a presentation highly atypical for EILO-glottic type),[17] which did not respond to reflux therapy or corticosteroids. She was successfully treated (based on visual description of postoperative laryngoscopy during deep inspiration) with carbon dioxide laser excision of redundant arytenoid mucosa as well as the corniculate and cuneiform cartilages.

SUPRAGLOTTOPLASTY AS A TREATMENT FOR EXERCISE-INDUCED LARYNGEAL OBSTRUCTION-SUPRAGLOTTIC TYPE: TECHNICAL CONSIDERATIONS

Supraglottoplasty is performed under general anesthesia by suspension laryngoscopy.[11] The laryngoscope is introduced to the vallecula and suspended in a position that exposes the aryepiglottic folds or epiglottis. The operating microscope improves visualization of the larynx. Technically the operation can be performed either by using surgical scissors or carbon dioxide laser.

The general aim of supraglottoplasty for EILO is to reduce supraglottic collapse with the rationale that this will improve inspiratory airflow through the larynx during exercise. In this procedure, surgeons increase the diameter of the laryngeal inlet (via elongation of the aryepiglottic folds, excision of redundant tissue, and possible rotation of the epiglottis toward the tongue base) and attempt to increase the structural integrity of the supraglottic structures. Specific anatomic decisions can be guided by findings on preoperative continuous laryngoscopy during exercise testing.

Elongation of the aryepiglottic folds is most often achieved by incisions in the upper rim of the aryepiglottic folds close to the lateral rim of the epiglottis, anteriorly to the corniculate tubercles. The incisions extend inferiorly to the superior border of the ventricular folds[11] (**Fig. 1**, Video 1). Reduction of excess tissue on the aryepiglottic folds, fixation of the epiglottis, or reduction of its size can be included in the operative procedure. Maat and colleagues[11] incised the aryepiglottic folds bilaterally close to the epiglottis and created a circular mucosa incision at the top of the corniculate tubercle to remove redundant mucosa.

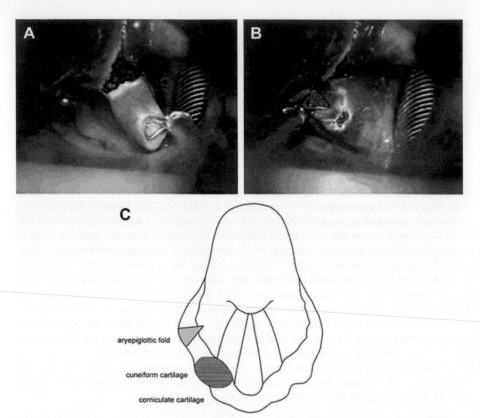

Fig. 1. Supraglottoplasty. (*A*) A CO$_2$ laser is used to make an incision in the aryepiglottic fold and (*B*) to remove the top of the cuneiforme (tubercle) cartilage and surrounding tissue. (*C*) Schematic drawing of the supraglottoplasty. (*From* Maat RC, Roksund OD, Olofsson J, et al. Surgical treatment of exercise-induced laryngeal dysfunction. Eur Arch Otorhinolaryngol 2007;264(4):403; with permission.)

SURGICAL INDICATIONS

At the current time, the indication for surgery in patients with refractory EILO is based solely on expert opinion. Maat and colleagues[7] proposed surgically treating patients with symptomatic EILO limited to the supraglottis. It is important that symptoms that are reported during CLE are similar in quality and quantity to field symptoms, because patients who do not fully reproduce symptoms in hospital settings may struggle with EILO that intermittently affects the glottis (which is likely unresponsive to surgical treatment).

It is the authors' opinion that surgery should be limited to patients with moderate or severe obstruction based on visual assessment and standardized scoring of CLE videos, because mild obstruction (slight inward rotation of the apex of the corniculate cartilage) may be a normal finding.[18] The authors recommend limiting surgery to those experiencing notable changes in quality of life attributable to the upper airway obstruction as defined by the patient. Finally, the authors recommend limiting surgery to patients who are fully informed of the potential risks and complications of this surgery and its irreversible nature. At the current time, given the series of limitations, surgery is likely to be limited to a few selected cases, with severe, refractory symptoms attributable to visualized supraglottic obstruction.

PUBLISHED OUTCOMES

Uncontrolled reports show a general trend indicating that surgery has a beneficial impact on EILO-related symptoms (**Table 2**). Maat and colleagues found that EILO patients reported fewer symptoms at 2- to 5-year follow-up than similar, conservatively treated patients using unvalidated symptom measures.[7] Supraglottoplasty seemed to have a lasting effect on EILO-related symptoms, and surgically treated patients were more physically active than nonsurgically treated patients with EILO at the time of follow-up. Mehlum and colleagues reported symptom improvement in surgically-treated patients in their follow-up study of 17 patients in 2016, using changes in visual analog scales of symptoms as a measure in an uncontrolled population.[13] Norlander and colleagues[12] reported improved symptom scores as rated by VAS and improved activity levels at the end of the follow-up period in surgically treated patients when compared with conservatively treated controls with EILO. Based on experience from these 48 patients treated with supraglottoplasty for EILO, the have preliminary data that suggest that the procedure is safe with effects lasting for several years.

Overall, although these reports are encouraging, overall assessment of surgical efficacy must be guarded. Analysis of the comparison studies is clearly confounded by selection bias, which likely leads to enrollment of highly motivated patients in groups that received surgery. Publication bias and reporting bias could theoretically enrich the literature with reports of successful cases. For this reason, the authors recommend surgery be reserved for highly selected cases with a frank and open discussion about the risks undertaken with any individual considering this approach to EILO treatment.

COMPLICATIONS

Analysis of medical literature on surgical complications in aggregate has revealed that supraglottoplasty is a safe procedure in neonates and children with CLM, as aspiration and airway stenosis are rare.[19] To the authors' knowledge no serious complications of supraglottoplasty in patients with EILO-supraglottic type have been reported. The 64 patients included in reports have to date not experienced serious adverse effects according to authors. However, long-term data with respect to complications related to aspiration are needed. The number of published procedures so far is limited and may underestimate rare complications. The authors recommend that surgeons publish complications or create surgical registries in order to assess rare procedural complications.

CURRENT CHALLENGES AND AREAS FOR FUTURE RESEARCH REGARDING SURGICAL MANAGEMENT OF EXERCISE-INDUCED LARYNGEAL OBSTRUCTION

There are several important issues to consider regarding the surgical treatment of EILO-supraglottic type. First, there are many unanswered questions related to

Table 2
The studies from Table 1 including pre-and post-operative evaluations with visual analogue scale (VAS) or CLE-score

Author, Year	Number	CLE score[18] Pre vs Post	Number	VAS Pre vs Post
Maat et al,[7] 2011	19	3.0 v.s. 1.7	23	90/30
Norlander et al,[12] 2015	0	—	14	8.2/3.8
Mehlum et al,[13] 2016	11	4.2 v.s. 3.2	11	78/33

disease mechanism. Is this a purely anatomic condition primarily affected by airway size, tissue pliability, and airflow? Are other factors equally important, including tissue reactivity, extrinsic triggers, breathing mechanics, and cognitive-behavioral factors? Are EILO-glottic type and EILO-supraglottic type part of the same disease spectrum, or are they separate entities with separate mechanisms? Some have hypothesized that supraglottic obstruction may cause glottic obstruction based on observations that have occurred across time in specific CLE examinations.[1] No specific data regarding mechanism of EILO-supraglottic type exist at the current time. This poor understanding of disease mechanism extends to a poor understanding of normal muscular function in the larynx during high-intensity exercise. Such an understanding is critical, as it will guide the development of future behavioral interventions as well as identification of specific surgical targets within the procedure.

Second, the specific location of surgical intervention within treatment algorithms is unclear. In reality, the role of surgery likely varies across centers in part because the availability and effectiveness of nonsurgical interventions (including speech-language pathology, inspiratory muscle training, and behavioral health consultations) also varies across centers. In order to address this challenge, the authors recommend standardization and assessment of nonsurgical interventions used in the treatment of EILO-supraglottic type. Inherent in this recommendation is identifying the need to quantitatively define normal function and quantitatively assess airway obstruction and symptom burden. Such quantitative assessment tools will also be useful in the assessment of surgical effectiveness.

Third, there are many unanswered questions regarding specific details of surgical technique during supraglottoplasty for EILO-supraglottic type. Although a general understanding of normal laryngeal function exists, the effect of supraglottoplasty for EILO on this function may be complicated. Which specific maneuvers within the surgery have the highest likelihood of improving symptoms and airflow? Which specific have the highest likelihood of increasing risk of complications? Are there maneuvers that can improve function without dramatically altering structure?

Finally, there are important questions about surgical outcomes. With fewer than 100 cases reported in the literature, none with follow-up reported into later life, it is reasonable to view surgery for EILO-supraglottic type cautiously. What percentage of patients improve to their baseline status postoperatively? Are there predictors of response to surgical intervention? Are there predictors of nonresponse? What are the long-term benefits and complications seen?

SUMMARY

Anatomic features of EILO-supraglottic type observed during CLE that resembled those seen in infants with CLM led to the extension of surgical interventions from CLM to patients with EILO-supraglottic type. Case reports and case controlled series of surgical interventions for this condition feature data that provide the rationale for future study of supraglottoplasty for refractory EILO-supraglottic type. Many unanswered questions remain regarding disease mechanism, indications for surgery, surgical technique, and outcomes. For these reasons, at the current time, the authors recommend consideration of supraglottoplasty only in patients with high impact, refractory symptoms clearly attributable to visualized EILO-supraglottic type who are clearly informed about the limited literature in the area, permanent nature of the procedure, and lack of long-term outcomes data.

SUPPLEMENTARY DATA

Supplementary data related to this article can be found online at https://doi.org/10.1016/j.iac.2018.01.005.

REFERENCES

1. Roksund OD, Maat RC, Heimdal JH, et al. Exercise induced dyspnea in the young. Larynx as the bottleneck of the airways. Respir Med 2009;103(12):1911–8.
2. Smith RJ, Bauman NM, Bent JP, et al. Exercise-induced laryngomalacia. Ann Otol Rhinol Laryngol 1995;104(7):537–41.
3. Christensen PM, Heimdal JH, Christopher KL, et al. ERS/ELS/ACCP 2013 international consensus conference nomenclature on inducible laryngeal obstructions. Eur Respir Rev 2015;24(137):445–50.
4. Thorne MC, Garetz SL. Laryngomalacia: review and summary of current clinical practice in 2015. Paediatr Respir Rev 2016;17:3–8.
5. Smith GJ, Cooper DM. Laryngomalacia and inspiratory obstruction in later childhood. Arch Dis Child 1981;56(5):345–9.
6. Richter GT, Rutter MJ, deAlarcon A, et al. Late-onset laryngomalacia: a variant of disease. Arch Otolaryngol Head Neck Surg 2008;134(1):75–80.
7. Maat RC, Hilland M, Roksund OD, et al. Exercise-induced laryngeal obstruction: natural history and effect of surgical treatment. Eur Arch Otorhinolaryngol 2011; 268(10):1485–92.
8. Gessler EM, Simko EJ, Greinwald JH Jr. Adult laryngomalacia: an uncommon clinical entity. Am J Otolaryngol 2002;23(6):386–9.
9. Siou GS, Jeannon JP, Stafford FW. Acquired idiopathic laryngomalacia treated by laser aryepiglottoplasty. J Laryngol Otol 2002;116(9):733–5.
10. Hilland M, Roksund OD, Sandvik L, et al. Congenital laryngomalacia is related to exercise-induced laryngeal obstruction in adolescence. Arch Dis Child 2016; 101(5):443–8.
11. Maat RC, Roksund OD, Olofsson J, et al. Surgical treatment of exercise-induced laryngeal dysfunction. Eur Arch Otorhinolaryngol 2007;264(4):401–7.
12. Norlander K, Johansson H, Jansson C, et al. Surgical treatment is effective in severe cases of exercise-induced laryngeal obstruction: a follow-up study. Acta Otolaryngol 2015;135(11):1152–9.
13. Mehlum CS, Walsted ES, Godballe C, et al. Supraglottoplasty as treatment of exercise induced laryngeal obstruction (EILO). Eur Arch Otorhinolaryngol 2016; 273(4):945–51.
14. Bent JP 3rd, Miller DA, Kim JW, et al. Pediatric exercise-induced laryngomalacia. Ann Otol Rhinol Laryngol 1996;105(3):169–75.
15. Björnsdóttir US, Gudmundsson K, Hjartarson H, et al. Exercise-induced laryngochalasia: an imitator of exercise-induced bronchospasm. Ann Allergy Asthma Immunol 2000;85(5):387–91.
16. Mandell DL, Arjmand EM. Laryngomalacia induced by exercise in a pediatric patient. Int J Pediatr Otorhinolaryngol 2003;67(9):999–1003.
17. Olin JT, Clary MS, Fan EM, et al. Continuous laryngoscopy quantitates laryngeal behaviour in exercise and recovery. Eur Respir J 2016;48(4): 1192–200.
18. Maat RC, Roksund OD, Halvorsen T, et al. Audiovisual assessment of exercise-induced laryngeal obstruction: reliability and validity of observations. Eur Arch Otorhinolaryngol 2009;266(12):1929–36.

19. Preciado D, Zalzal G. A systematic review of supraglottoplasty outcomes. Arch Otolaryngol Head Neck Surg 2012;138(8):718–21.
20. Chemery L, Le Clech G, Delaval P, et al. Exercise-induced laryngomalacia. Rev Mal Respir 2002;19:641–3.

Exertional Dyspnea and Excessive Dynamic Airway Collapse

Michael J. Morris, MD*, Jeffrey T. Woods, MD,
Cameron W. McLaughlin, DO

KEYWORDS

- Dyspnea • Exercise • Excessive dynamic airway collapse • Tracheobronchomalacia
- Asthma • Chronic obstructive pulmonary disease

KEY POINTS

- Excessive dynamic airway collapse (EDAC), which is functional large airway collapse, can occur during exercise.
- EDAC symptoms include exertional dyspnea and centralized expiratory wheezing.
- EDAC may be identified in patients with chronic obstructive pulmonary disease or asthma.

INTRODUCTION

Excessive dynamic airway collapse (EDAC) is a recent term applied to individuals identified with functional collapse of the large airways. It is generally defined as excessive bulging of the posterior tracheal membrane into the airway lumen (usually >75%) during expiration without cartilage collapse to distinguish this entity from tracheobronchomalacia (TBM).[1] It has been primarily associated with underlying airway disorders, such as chronic obstructive pulmonary disease (COPD), asthma, and bronchiectasis.[2] Those patients with moderate to severe symptoms can present with cough, wheezing, dyspnea, or recurrent respiratory infections related to exacerbations of their lung disease. Likewise, it may become symptomatic after mild to moderate exertion. Current guidelines suggest that functional status (exertion, daily activities, or rest), length of

The view(s) expressed herein are those of the author(s) and do not reflect the official policy or position of Brooke Army Medical Center, the US Army Medical Department, the US Army Office of the Surgeon General, the Department of the Army, the Department of the Air Force, Department of Defense, or the US Government.

Dr M.J. Morris is a paid speaker for Janssen Pharmaceuticals.

Pulmonary/Critical Care Service (MCHE-ZMD-P), Department of Medicine, San Antonio Military Medical Center, 3551 Roger Brooke Drive, JBSA Fort Sam Houston, TX 78234, USA

* Corresponding author. Pulmonary Disease Service (MCHE-ZDM-P), San Antonio Military Medical Center, 3551 Roger Brooke Drive, JBSA Fort Sam Houston, TX 78234.

E-mail address: michael.j.morris34.civ@mail.mil

Immunol Allergy Clin N Am 38 (2018) 325–332
https://doi.org/10.1016/j.iac.2018.01.006
0889-8561/18/Published by Elsevier Inc.

immunology.theclinics.com

the tracheobronchial wall affected, and severity of collapse are also important to define in patients diagnosed with EDAC.[2]

Much of the description of EDAC has focused on exacerbations of underlying disease with little discussion on its relationship to exercise. Weinstein and colleagues[3] recently published a case series of 6 individuals in the military with symptomatic EDAC only during exercise. All had exertional symptoms, expiratory wheezing, and confirmed visual evidence of large airway collapse (>75%) with fiberoptic bronchoscopy (FOB). The findings have expanded the differential in the challenging evaluation of exertional dyspnea patients with otherwise normal pulmonary function testing (PFT) and chest imaging.[4] In this review, the authors aim to discuss the relationship between exercise and EDAC and further elucidate its potential impact on exercise limitation.

EXCESSIVE DYNAMIC AIRWAY COLLAPSE DEFINITION

EDAC is generally defined as excessive bulging of the posterior tracheal membrane during expiration with greater than 75% collapse of the airway lumen. It is distinctly different from TBM because of the absence of cartilaginous involvement. These distinct clinical entities may be very similar in presentation and have been referred to collectively as expiratory central airway collapse.[2] However, there is no universally accepted cutoff value to separate normal from abnormal expiratory airway narrowing, but generally greater than 75% closure of the airway lumen has been suggested to be clinically important.

Reflecting tidal cycling of intrathoracic pressure, there is inward bulging of the posterior membrane of the trachea and main bronchi that occurs normally during exhalation. This airway compression, known as dynamic airway collapse, can ordinarily narrow the lumen of normal central airways by up to 50%. Posterior membrane collapse has also been described to be partly physiologic and associated with forced expiration or cough. Defining the clinical significance of EDAC can be problematic as functional airway collapse in healthy individuals has been documented. There is a wide variation in bronchial collapse with forced expiration on multidetector computed tomographic (CT) imaging in healthy volunteers with normal PFT and no significant smoke exposure.[5,6]

PATHOPHYSIOLOGY

It is currently theorized that large airway collapse related to EDAC is due to increased airway resistance distal to the equal pressure point, decreased lung elastic recoil, and increased pleural pressures. During exercise itself, there is increased luminal airflow velocity leading to a decrease in luminal pressures, especially in tapering airways, and creating a stress on luminal integrity with subsequent smooth muscle fatigue or strain. This muscle lassitude in the setting of continued pressure differential is the likely culprit for why this change in airway diameter is not identified on nonexertional pulmonary testing.[7]

The pathogenesis of EDAC has been described as being a result of 2 primary circumstances. One factor is weakening of the smooth muscle tone of the posterior membrane. The other factor is a decrease in luminal pressures in regions of tapering airways (Bernoulli's principle) in the setting of reduced elastic recoil, thus creating even greater narrowing leading to greater transmural pressure gradient.[8] The diagnosis of EDAC has primarily been described in patients with underlying lung disorders such as COPD or asthma, especially in those patients with identifiable TBM. The underlying lung pathology likely contributes to the chronic atrophy and strain of longitudinal smooth muscle given the excessive airway pressure gradients typically seen in these disease processes.[9]

EDAC as seen on FOB or dynamic chest CT imaging occurs at the compressible segment of the central airway proximal to the equal pressure point. Likewise, tracheal collapse is caused by increased airway resistance distal to the equal pressure point, decreased lung elastic recoil, and increased pleural pressure. This mechanism explains the finding of EDAC in patients with uncontrolled asthma, COPD, and obesity, especially when 2 or more of those disorders coexist.[10] When EDAC is defined as a forced expiratory collapse of greater than 80% of the airway lumen, there is no significant correlation between end-expiratory or dynamic expiratory collapse and percent predicted forced expiratory volume at 1 second (FEV_1).[7] Consistent with the hypothesis that EDAC is typically a consequence of peripheral airway disorders and not central airway pathology, there is documented improvement in EDAC after lung transplantation or lung volume reduction surgery in patients with emphysema. However, the mechanism in patients without underlying lung pathology as described by Weinstein and colleagues[3] has not been elucidated.

EXCESSIVE DYNAMIC AIRWAY COLLAPSE IN CHRONIC OBSTRUCTIVE PULMONARY DISEASE AND ASTHMA

EDAC is most often associated with COPD. The largest study documenting the prevalence of EDAC in COPD described an overall prevalence of 6% in COPD patients.[11] Prior studies have demonstrated an EDAC prevalence from 9% to 22% in COPD.[10,12–15] The definition used for EDAC varied across the studies, with a greater than 50% to 80% decrease in cross-sectional area (CSA) used. In addition, the methods used to identify EDAC were not uniform and included FOB, dynamic CT scan, and end-expiratory CT imaging. In COPD patients, EDAC is associated with a higher GOLD (Global Initiative for Chronic Obstructive Lung Disease) stage, increased airflow limitation on spirometry, worsened dyspnea scores, and increased frequency of severe COPD.[11] EDAC has also been implicated as a potential cause of persistent wheezing in COPD patients; up to 40% with persistent wheezing have been found to have EDAC.[16]

An increased body mass index (BMI) is also associated with an increased prevalence of EDAC in COPD. Two studies found a statistically significant association with BMI; both studies evaluated COPD patients and found that a higher BMI, greater than 30 and 35, were linked with the finding of EDAC.[11,17] Furthermore, there was not an association with BMI and EDAC in those patients without COPD.[17] Whether EDAC causes clinically important flow limitation remains a subject of current debate. In a recent study of patients with COPD, no significant correlation was observed between the degree of static end-expiratory or dynamic forced expiratory tracheal collapse and FEV_1 percent predicted.[10] However, a secondary analysis of patients enrolled in the US National Institutes of Health COPD Gene study did reveal an adverse association between EDAC and quality of life as measured by the St George's Respiratory Questionnaire (SGRQ).[11]

Most of the evidence linking asthma with EDAC is in the form of case reports of difficult-to-control asthma with subsequent identification of EDAC.[18,19] One study has prospectively evaluated 202 asthmatic patients with FOB and identified a prevalence of 31%, noting that the EDAC prevalence increased with the severity of asthma.[20] There are no available data regarding the impact of EDAC on asthma exacerbations, quality-of-life scores, or exertional symptoms. In addition, it is unclear from the published data whether the cases presented truly have asthma or if EDAC is the primary underlying cause merely mimicking asthma.[18,19]

EXCESSIVE DYNAMIC AIRWAY COLLAPSE AND FUNCTIONAL CAPACITY

The impact of EDAC itself on functional capacity is unknown because most of the data are derived from the COPD population. In the largest cohort of EDAC patients, it was demonstrated that EDAC leads to increased dyspnea and poorer respiratory quality of life, but there was no impact on 6-minute walk testing (6MWT).[11] In addition, a small series of both EDAC and TBM patients (n = 18) who underwent airway stenting identified that half had improvement in their modified World Health Organization (WHO) functional classification.[21] In this study, patients with the more severe cases showed improvement, whereas the milder cases did not. Boiselle and colleagues[12] studied 100 COPD patients with full PFTs, 6MWT, SGRQ, and dynamic CT scanning. Twenty percent of the patients were identified with expiratory collapse based on greater than 80% expiratory reduction in the tracheal lumen CSA during the expiration phase of CT scanning. This study was unable to identify differences in FEV_1, diffusing capacity, 6MWT, or SGRQ activity scores between COPD patients without and with excessive tracheal collapse, respectively. Represas-Represas and colleagues[15] studied 53 COPD patients with collapse at different levels by dynamic CT imaging and did not demonstrate differences in Medical Research Council dyspnea index scores or 6MWT.

EXERCISE-ASSOCIATED EXCESSIVE DYNAMIC AIRWAY COLLAPSE

Weinstein and colleagues[3] published a unique case series of 6 patients identified during comprehensive evaluation for post–deployment respiratory symptoms. Most notably, this group of patients reported symptoms of audible "wheezing" with exertional dyspnea. None of the patients were found to have evidence of underlying obstructive or interstitial lung disease. High-resolution computed tomography (HRCT) was notable for significant expiratory collapse in 2 patients, whereas dynamic CT demonstrated collapse in an additional 2 patients. Four of the patients had audible expiratory large airway wheezing that developed during exercise (not present at rest) with further localization by chest auscultation, and the 2 remaining patients had expiratory wheezing localized only by auscultation. Flexible bronchoscopy was able to localize the site of obstruction (>75% obstruction of the affected airway) that corresponded directly to the auscultatory findings. This included 2 patients who underwent awake exercise FOB used to identify the site of obstruction (see video file from Weinstein and colleagues[3]). These 6 individuals were identified with exercise-associated EDAC using the following criteria:

1. Exertional dyspnea without resting symptoms,
2. Focal expiratory wheezing during exercise,
3. Functional collapse of the large airways during FOB,
4. Expiratory CT imaging with narrowing of the airway, and
5. Absence of underlying pulmonary pathology.[3]

EXCESSIVE DYNAMIC AIRWAY COLLAPSE EVALUATION

In most EDAC patients, typical symptoms may include chronic cough, dyspnea, wheezing, stridor, orthopnea, recurrent pulmonary infections, and impaired clearance of respiratory secretions. These symptoms may be triggered by numerous factors to include upper respiratory infections, dust exposure, exercise, recumbent positioning, forced exhalation, and cough.[11,18,20,22,23] Immediate onset of dyspnea with exertion may differentiate EDAC from COPD and asthma, whereby symptom onset with exertion may be more gradual.[19] An initial step in identifying EDAC in any given patient is careful physical examination, which may identify and localize airway sounds that are directly emanating from the large airways. Localization of an expiratory wheeze (which may be heard in all lung fields) to the central airways should prompt a clinician to further investigate. In patients identified with exercise-associated EDAC, this finding on lung examination prompted further imaging studies. This included either HRCT with expiratory images or a dynamic CT in which the patient actively performs a forced expiratory maneuver. In individuals with exertional symptoms, performing some type of exercise study may cause EDAC and wheezing not present at rest. Another important step in eliminating other causes is performance of exercise laryngoscopy to rule out laryngeal disorders, such as inducible laryngeal obstruction.[24]

AIRWAY IMAGING (DYNAMIC COMPUTED TOMOGRAPHY)

Airway imaging in EDAC may demonstrate a significant change in the luminal CRA of the airway in the inspiratory and expiratory phases as demonstrated in numerous studies.[1,11,12,23,25,26] CT imaging during inspiratory and expiratory phases may demonstrate dynamic collapse of the trachea and main bronchi during the expiratory phase with posterior membrane bulging, in contrast to TBM, which is associated with anterolateral wall collapse.[18,25,27] Dynamic CT is the preferred imaging modality over static imaging, because the latter may lessen the degree of airway collapse.[2] Dynamic CT may be equal to FOB in the diagnosis of EDAC, providing an important noninvasive method of diagnosis.[1,8,28] Although CSA narrowing greater than 50% is typically used to define EDAC for research purposes, there are data that normal individuals may have a 35% decrease in CSA, and one study of healthy volunteers found 78% of participants exceeded greater than 50% decrease in CSA.[5,6]

FUNCTIONAL BRONCHOSCOPY

Fiberoptic bronchoscopy should be performed in all patients suspected of having EDAC to identify the presence or absence of EDAC and determination of the site of obstruction.[8,18,29,30] Suggested specific indications for functional bronchoscopy are shown in **Box 1**. If possible, sedation should be minimized to allow the patient to follow commands to better demonstrate airway abnormalities associated with the inspiratory and expiratory phases. Fiberoptic bronchoscopy in EDAC may demonstrate narrowing of the airway lumen with expiratory maneuvers and more commonly with cough.[13,23] One study evaluating estimates of the degree of airway collapse during FOB found high interoperator and intraoperator reliability, supporting the use of FOB in the diagnosis of EDAC.[9] The use of endobronchial ultrasound in EDAC may

---

Box 1
Indications for functional bronchoscopy

1. Audible wheezing caused by exercise

2. Wheezing that localizes to the large airways on clinical examination

3. Concern for tracheobronchomalacia

4. Evidence of large airway collapse identified by CT scanning

5. Recurrent COPD or asthma exacerbations

6. Persistent wheezing despite treatment

7. Unexplained dyspnea after noninvasive evaluation

demonstrate normal anterior cartilaginous structures and thin posterior membrane.[21] Findings consistent with EDAC may be evident in 5% to 23% of patients undergoing FOB for undifferentiated respiratory symptoms, and common findings include chronic inflammation, lymphocytic predominance, and negative cultures.[22,25] In selected individuals with symptoms at higher levels of exercise, awake FOB during exercise (typically cycle ergometry) with the onset of symptoms was shown to be diagnostic.[3]

TREATMENT OPTIONS

Currently, there are few treatment options available to those patients identified with EDAC. Therapy primarily should center on treating the underlying disease process (COPD, asthma, bronchiectasis) to limit the number and frequency of exacerbations. Each exacerbation with resultant increases in wheezing, cough, and airway secretions may intensify the sensation of dyspnea because of increases in airway collapse. Primary treatment modalities for both TBM and EDAC also include the use of noninvasive positive pressure ventilation (NIPPV) to prevent large airway collapse. NIPPV functions to open the large airways and decrease the work of breathing, aiding in drainage of respiratory secretions and possibly improving nocturnal wheezing; it does not improve dyspnea and cough.[1,23] Seven to 10 cm of water pressure is typically sufficient to increase intraluminal pressure, lung volumes, and elastic recoil and may be titrated during functional FOB.[2,7] It is likewise important to screen for obstructive sleep apnea in patients with EDAC who require NIPPV.[8] Notably, there is an ongoing study currently being conducted to evaluate daytime use of continuous positive airway pressure (CPAP) in patients with tracheomalacia.[31]

The use of mechanical airway stenting and possible tracheobronchoplasty is reserved for selected individuals with EDAC with severe symptoms and a significant limitation in overall functional classification (class III or IV).[1,10] As described in several studies of patients with severe TBM, improvement of respiratory symptoms, quality of life, and WHO functional class occurred after airway stenting and/or surgical intervention in selected candidates.[9,32] Aggressive interventions for EDAC are generally preferred only for cases refractory to conservative management and NIPPV whereby the potential benefit of the invasive procedure outweighs the associated risk.[7]

For EDAC symptoms related specifically to exercise, treatment options are very limited. It is not recommended for these patients to undergo airway stenting or tracheobronchoplasty based on the impact of disease. The authors have recommended to their patients with exercise-associated EDAC to limit exertional activities (running, jogging, and so forth) to a less strenuous pace or distance where symptoms such as dyspnea and audible wheezing are minimized. In this group of patients, reduction in exercise has been adequate to control their symptoms. In addition, consideration should be given for CPAP use if symptomatic at rest or after exercise.[31] It is not known whether continued exercise will worsen the extent or severity of EDAC in this group of patients. Notably, several of the active duty military patients had to leave the military given their limitations with aerobic activity.

SUMMARY

EDAC (with or without underlying lung disease) is very likely aggravated by exercise and may be symptom limiting in many individuals. Given the increases in minute ventilation during exercise, increased flows are likely to make airway collapse more pronounced. Careful evaluation should be undertaken to identify patients with EDAC and its contribution to airway symptoms during exercise. Use of dynamic CT imaging or FOB should help to identify patients with underlying EDAC and potentially alter treatment plans. Future priorities for defining this entity are as follows:

1. To more fully describe the role of exertional EDAC in patients with asthma through use of exercise bronchoscopy and
2. Increase the utilization of dynamic CT imaging and functional bronchoscopy in suspected large airway collapse.

REFERENCES

1. Murgu SD, Colt HG. Tracheobronchomalacia and excessive dynamic airway collapse. Respirology 2006;11(4):388–406.
2. Murgu S, Colt H. Tracheobronchomalacia and excessive dynamic airway collapse. Clin Chest Med 2013;34(3):527–55.
3. Weinstein DJ, Hull JE, Ritchie BL, et al. Exercise-associated excessive dynamic airway collapse in military personnel. Ann Am Thorac Soc 2016;13(9):1476–82.
4. Morris MJ, Grbach VX, Deal LE, et al. Evaluation of exertional dyspnea in the active duty patient: the diagnostic approach and the utility of clinical testing. Mil Med 2002;167(4):281–8.
5. Boiselle PM, O'Donnell CR, Bankier AA, et al. Tracheal collapsibility in healthy volunteers during forced expiration: assessment with multidetector CT. Radiology 2009;252(1):255–62.
6. O'Donnell CR, Litmanovich D, Loring SH, et al. Age and sex dependence of forced expiratory central airway collapse in healthy volunteers. Chest 2012; 142(1):168–74.
7. Murgu S, Stoy S. Excessive dynamic airway collapse: a standalone cause of exertional dyspnea? Ann Am Thorac Soc 2016;13(9):1437–9.
8. Kalra A, Abouzgheib W, Gajera M, et al. Excessive dynamic airway collapse for the internist: new nomenclature or different entity? Postgrad Med J 2011; 87(1029):482–6.
9. Majid A, Gaurav K, Sanchez JM, et al. Evaluation of tracheobronchomalacia by dynamic flexible bronchoscopy. A pilot study. Ann Am Thorac Soc 2014;11(6): 951–5.
10. O'Donnell CR, Bankier AA, O'Donnell DH, et al. Static end-expiratory and dynamic forced expiratory tracheal collapse in COPD. Clin Radiol 2014;69(4): 357–62.
11. Bhatt SP, Terry NLJ, Nath H, et al. Association between expiratory central airway collapse and respiratory outcomes among smokers. JAMA 2016;315(5):498–505.
12. Boiselle PM, Michaud G, Roberts DH, et al. Dynamic expiratory tracheal collapse in COPD. Correlation with clinical and physiologic parameters. Chest 2012; 142(6):1539–44.
13. Ellingsen I, Holmedahl NH. Does excessive dynamic airway collapse have any impact on dynamic pulmonary function tests? J Bronchology Interv Pulmonol 2014;21(1):40–6.
14. Ochs RA, Petkovska I, Kim HJ, et al. Prevalence of tracheal collapse in an emphysema cohort as measured with end-expiration CT. Acad Radiol 2009; 16(1):46–53.
15. Represas-Represas C, Leiro-Fernández V, Mallo-Alonso R, et al. Excessive dynamic airway collapse in a small cohort of chronic obstructive pulmonary disease patients. Ann Thorac Med 2015;10(2):118–22.

16. Sindhwani G, Sodhi R, Saini M, et al. Tracheobronchomalacia/excessive dynamic airway collapse in patients with chronic obstructive pulmonary disease with persistent expiratory wheeze: a pilot study. Lung India 2016;33(4):381.

17. Boiselle PM, Litmanovich DE, Michaud G, et al. Dynamic expiratory tracheal collapse in morbidly obese COPD patients. COPD 2013;10(5):604–10.

18. Behazin N, Jones SB, Cohen RI, et al. Respiratory restriction and elevated pleural and esophageal pressures in morbid obesity. J Appl Physiol (1985) 2010;108(1): 212–8.

19. Harada Y, Kondo T. Excessive dynamic airway collapse detected using nondynamic CT. Intern Med 2016;55(11):1477–9.

20. Hunter JH, Stanford W, Smith JM, et al. Expiratory collapse of the trachea presenting as worsening asthma. Chest 1993;104(2):633–5.

21. Dal Negro RW, Tognella S, Guerriero M, et al. Prevalence of tracheobronchomalacia and excessive dynamic airway collapse in bronchial asthma of different severity. Multidiscip Respir Med 2013;8(1):32.

22. Murgu SD, Colt HG. Description of a multidimensional classification system for patients with expiratory central airway collapse. Respirology 2007;12(4):543–50.

23. Bozoghlanian V, Williams SJ, Ismail H, et al. Dynamic airway collapse: a frequently misdiagnosed asthma mimicker. Ann Allergy Asthma Immunol 2016; 116(1):87–8.

24. Choo EM, Seaman JC, Musani AI. Tracheomalacia/tracheobronchomalacia and hyperdynamic airway collapse. Immunol Allergy Clin N Am 2013;33(1):23–34.

25. Morris MJ, Christopher KL. Diagnostic criteria for the classification of vocal cord dysfunction. Chest 2010;138(5):1213–22.

26. Handa H, Miyazawa T, Murgu SD, et al. Novel multimodality imaging and physiologic assessments clarify choke-point physiology and airway wall structure in expiratory central airway collapse. Respir Care 2012;57(4):634–41.

27. Joosten S, MacDonald M, Lau KK, et al. Excessive dynamic airway collapse comorbid with COPD diagnosed using 320-slice dynamic CT scanning technology. Thorax 2012;67(1):95–6.

28. Matus I, Richter W, Mani SB. Awareness, competencies, and practice patterns in tracheobronchomalacia: a survey of pulmonologists. J Bronchology Interv Pulmonol 2016;23(2):131–7.

29. Kauczor HU, Wielpütz MO, Owsijewitsch M, et al. Computed tomographic imaging of the airways in COPD and asthma. J Thorac Imaging 2011;26(4):290–300.

30. Bardin PG, Johnston SL, Hamilton G. Middle airway obstruction – it may be happening under our noses. Thorax 2013;68:396–8.

31. Patout M, Mylott L, Kent R, et al. Trial of portable continuous positive airway pressure for the management of tracheobronchomalacia. Am J Respir Crit Care Med 2016;193(10):e57.

32. Ernst A, Odell DD, Michaud G, et al. Central airway stabilization for tracheobronchomalacia improves quality of life in patients with COPD. Chest 2011;140(5): 1162–8.

The Future of Exertional Respiratory Problems

What Do We Know About the Total Airway Approach and What Do We Need to Know?

J. Tod Olin, MD, MSCS[a],*, James H. Hull, MD, PhD[b]

KEYWORDS

- Exertional dyspnea • Exercise-induced laryngeal obstruction
- Excessive dynamic airway collapse • Exercise-induced bronchoconstriction

KEY POINTS

- Exercise is increasingly viewed as a preventative and therapeutic modality for a variety of medical and behavioral health disorders; therefore, it is imperative to minimize barriers that discourage exercise.
- This issue of *Immunology and Allergy Clinics of North America* details a "total airway approach" to the evaluation of exertional respiratory problems.
- This issue focuses on basic elements of 2 of sinonasal disease and excessive dynamic airway collapse; more complicated considerations are discussed with respect to exercise-induced laryngeal obstruction.
- A rigorous discussion of the mechanisms, diagnostics, and therapeutics for exercise-induced bronchoconstriction follows, reflective of more than 5 decades of research in the area.
- There is much room for growth in research in these areas, and in common inflammatory pathways and neurophysiologic coupling across all airway segments.

THE IMPORTANCE OF A TOTAL AIRWAY APPROACH TO EXERTIONAL DYSPNEA

In an age when exercise is viewed as a preventative or therapeutic modality for a variety of medical and behavioral health conditions, it is imperative that the medical, surgical, and behavioral health communities minimize barriers that discourage patients from exercising.[1] Exertional respiratory symptoms such as dyspnea, cough, and wheeze represent some of the most important problems acting as such a barrier faced by patients of general practitioners, allergists/immunologists, pulmonologists,

[a] Department of Pediatrics, Division of Pediatric Pulmonology, Pediatric Exercise Tolerance Center, National Jewish Health, 1400 Jackson Street, Denver, CO 80206, USA; [b] Department of Respiratory Medicine, Royal Brompton Hospital, Fulham Road, SW3 6HP, London, UK
* Corresponding author.
E-mail address: olint@njhealth.org

Immunol Allergy Clin N Am 38 (2018) 333–339
https://doi.org/10.1016/j.iac.2018.01.013
0889-8561/18/© 2018 Elsevier Inc. All rights reserved.

otolaryngologists, and cardiologists. This collection of reviews has highlighted the history and recent improvements in our understanding of exertional symptoms attributable to the airway. The primary goal of this edition was to introduce a conceptual framework for clinicians to use in the approach to exertional respiratory problems, championing a "total airway" approach.

A secondary goal of this issue is to identify areas for growth in our scientific understanding of specific causes of exertional dyspnea attributable to the airway. Clearly, the medical and research communities have appreciated the impact of asthma during exercise for decades.[2] We propose the total airway approach as a conceptual framework for contextualizing asthma research as well as research devoted to sinonasal disease, the larynx, and the central airways.[3–5] Using this framework, gaps in scientific knowledge become more apparent.

TOTAL AIRWAY APPROACH: WHAT DO WE KNOW?

From a clinical perspective, the collective expertise of the immunology/allergy, pulmonology, otolaryngology, speech-language pathology, and psychology communities featured in this edition can be pooled to develop diagnostic and treatment suggestions for providers of patients with exertional dyspnea. Although formal multidisciplinary teams are sparse, an appreciation of the multidisciplinary nature of exertional respiratory problems may lead to a more thoughtful approach by all providers.

In this issue, we began by discussing interactions between exercise and sinonasal disease (see Brecht Steelant and colleagues' article, "Exercise and Sino-Nasal Disease," in this issue). This is a field in its infancy and rarely discussed in the literature despite the very high prevalence of sinonasal disease in the general population and increased prevalence among elite athletes.[6] Seys and colleagues highlight some of the cellular mechanisms and physiologic consequences known to be involved in disease as well as the diagnostic and therapeutic options available to clinicians.

This issue of the *Immunology and Allergy Clinics of North America* is replete with a number of reviews (articles 2 through 6) devoted to exercise-induced laryngeal obstruction (EILO), which, since its initial recognition as a cause of exertional dyspnea in the 1980s, is increasingly recognized as an important cause of exertional dyspnea in specific populations.[7] In the second article, Walsted and colleagues (see Leif Nordang and colleagues' article, "Exercise Induced Laryngeal Obstruction – An Overview," in this issue) taught us that that its prevalence lies in the 5% to 10% range in select demographic groups and societies, which is a prevalence comparable with that of asthma in the general population, and yet it remains almost completely unrecognized and certainly misdiagnosed in clinical practice.[8,9] It may be completely distinct from inducible laryngeal obstruction caused by other triggers at rest, the condition described by Dunglison, Patterson, and Christopher, which has been described with many names including vocal cord dysfunction and paradoxic vocal fold motion.[10–12] Halvorsen and colleagues (see Ola Drange Røksund and colleagues' article, "Working Towards a Common Transatlantic Approach for Evaluation of Exercise Induced Laryngeal Obstruction," in this issue) described a variety of invasive and noninvasive diagnostic techniques that have been used in the past few decades, and noted that continuous laryngoscopy during exercise is emerging as the preferred diagnostic method for its ability to contextualize partial airway obstruction in relation to symptoms of interest, exercise intensity, and recovery.[13,14] A variety of medical, behavioral, and surgical approaches to treatment have been proposed, each with potential benefits and shortcomings. Bergevin and colleagues (see Monica Shaffer and colleagues' article, "Speech-Language Pathology as a Primary Treatment for

Exercise-Induced Laryngeal Obstruction (EILO)," in this issue) provide a detailed summary of speech-language pathology interventions that have been published since the 1980s.[12,15] Olin and colleagues and Heimdal and colleagues (see J. Tod Olin and Erika Westhoff (Carlson)'s article, "Exercise-Induced Laryngeal Obstruction and Performance Psychology: Using the Mind as a Diagnostic and Therapeutic Target"; and see John-Helge Heimdal and colleagues' article, "Surgical Intervention for Exercise-Induced Laryngeal Obstruction," in this issue) follow with a summary of available therapeutic knowledge in the behavioral health and surgical realms respectively, fields in their infancy, ripe for future research.[16–18]

Next, excessive dynamic airway collapse (EDAC) is covered, a condition only recently described as a potential cause of exertional dyspnea (see Michael J. Morris and colleagues' article, "Exertional Dyspnea and Excessive Dynamic Airway Collapse," in this issue).[5,19] Morris and colleagues taught us about the proposed physiology, presentation, and clinical relevance of the condition. Importantly, we present a discussion about this clinical entity in the context of our existing knowledge of tracheobronchomalacia. Finally, diagnostic and therapeutic approaches are proposed, although there is limited evidence to dictate whether they are truly robust or beneficial.

To complete the issue, a series of reviews (articles 8 through 13) cover exercise-induced bronchoconstriction with asthma and exercise-induced bronchoconstriction without asthma, conditions that have been the primary focus of airway literature both clinically and scientifically for the past several decades.[20] Bonini and Silvers (see Matteo Bonini and William Silvers' article, "Exercise-Induced Bronchoconstriction: Background, Prevalence and Sport Considerations," in this issue) discuss the effect of different sports on the prevalence of these conditions.[21] Kippelen and colleagues (see Pascale Kippelen and colleagues' article, "Mechanisms and Biomarkers of Exercise-Induced Bronchoconstriction," in this issue) synthesize an incredible review of decades of mechanistic research in EIB, incorporating observations attributable to vascular phenomena into the now accepted osmotic hypothesis.[22,23] In addition to cellular mechanisms, newer neurogenic mechanisms of disease are discussed. Rundell and colleagues (see Kenneth W. Rundell and colleagues' article, "Exercise-Induced Bronchoconstriction and the Air We breathe," in this issue) followed with one of the most comprehensive reviews of interactions between asthma and the environment available, featuring knowledge on many commonly encountered environmental pollutants. Brannan and colleagues (see John D. Brannan and Celeste Porsbjerg's article, "Testing for Exercise Induced-Bronchoconstriction," in this issue) discussed the latest advances in EIB diagnosis, highlighting the practical and physiologic advantages of surrogate testing.[24] Backer and Mastronarde (see Vibeke Backer and John Mastronarde's article, "Pharmacologic Strategies for Exercise-Induced Bronchospasm with a focus on Athletes," in this issue) provide a comprehensive summary of pharmacologic options for clinicians, incorporating guidelines from the American Thoracic Society, American Academy of Allergy, Asthma, and Immunology, and American College of Allergy, Asthma and Immunology.[20,25] Finally, Dickinson and colleagues (see John Dickinson and colleagues' article, "Non-Pharmacological Strategies to Manage Exercise Induced Bronchoconstriction," in this issue) discussed several nonpharmacologic interventions for EIB, a topic of keen interest to many athletes.

TOTAL AIRWAY APPROACH: WHAT DO WE NEED TO KNOW?

This issue of *Immunology and Allergy Clinics of North America* has identified potential areas of immediate impact for potential future research across the airway. Our understanding of diseases localized to specific locations in the airway varies greatly by location. With respect to other diseases of the airway, our understanding of lower airways disease is relatively sophisticated. Lower airways disease is increasingly understood to be a syndrome of clinical symptoms that occur as a final common pathway to a variety of insulted and dysregulated molecular and cellular pathways. On the other extreme, sinonasal disease, EILO and EDAC are poorly understood from the gross perspectives of mechanisms, physiology, and clinical impact. Moreover, there are currently no high-quality studies (ie, with a randomized, controlled intervention) assessing treatment in these areas.

With respect to understanding interactions between nasal processes and exercise, there are several clinical questions that require answering in the coming years. In the short term, it is critical to characterize the impact of nasal symptoms on exertional dyspnea as a whole. A functional assay of nasal air flow function could enable clinicians to quantitate nasal function, define threshold levels for abnormalities, and measure response to therapy. Such an assay could characterize the impact of changes in nasal flow on dyspnea more broadly.

From a more basic perspective, it will be helpful to understand the molecular and cellular mechanisms that lead to airflow obstruction. This understanding could help to characterize the effect of exercise on epithelial stress and nasal obstruction more broadly. Moreover, such an understanding will lead to understanding of the relative effects of various exercise modes on nasal function.

Turning to EILO, the publication of this issue coincides with the timing of the first international meeting of clinicians and researchers focused on EILO, in Bergen, Norway. The proceedings of this meeting featured focused discussion on available diagnostic and therapeutic strategies and serve as a useful guide to the identification of clinical and research gaps. Although there was broad consensus that continuous laryngoscopy during exercise is the diagnostic approach of choice among meeting participants, there is a need to reach agreement on protocols and exercise modalities used to provoke field symptoms, especially for the standardization of research protocols. There is a need to correlate observed upper airway obstruction and physiologic variables of clinical significance to define threshold levels of obstruction that define disease. The meeting participants agreed that there was an urgent need for a system that permits quantification of observed obstruction beyond the existing semiquantitative measures. There is also a need for a robust clinical outcome measure that is specific to exercise.

Beyond the immediate clinical gaps noted in EILO, it is notable that disease mechanism is poorly understood at the current time. It is not clear if EILO is a singular entity or a syndrome of related phenomena. The relative impact of absolute airway size, airway pliability, airway reactivity, extrinsic contributors (allergic rhinitis and gastroesophageal reflux), cortical processes and motor learning are currently unknown.

With respect to EDAC, active research is just beginning, and many clinical questions remain unanswered. From an applied clinical perspective, we do not have precise diagnostic techniques. For this reason, estimates of prevalence and characterizations of normal function are not available. The correlation of obstruction and symptoms is not clear at the current time and, thus, the importance of the phenomenon is not clear. Treatment remains quite a mystery, especially in light of the uncertainty as to whether this is a primary or secondary phenomenon. Symptom-based outcome measures could guide this process. On a similar note, from a more basic perspective, the disease mechanism must be elucidated somewhat moving forward if progress is to be achieved. Such knowledge could potentially lead to preventative strategies.

Finally, EIB presents a number of questions as well, albeit at a more refined level. Clinically, with our improved understanding of disease mechanism, it is reasonable to wonder whether more precise therapeutic targets a possibility, analogous to the newer biologic agents available for refractory asthma. The true interaction between nonpharmacologic and pharmacologic interventions remain to be defined. There is also a need to study pharmacologic and nonpharmacologic interventions that protect athletes from noxious environmental stimuli and associated airway injury, with an eye toward disease prevention.

THE FUTURE OF "TOTAL AIRWAY" RESEARCH

Research devoted to specific causes of exertional dyspnea attributable to the airway will lead to increasingly precise characterization and treatment for patients in the future. However, a total airway approach will elucidate the mechanistic, physiologic, and clinical impact of interactions between conditions.

How does the inflammatory biology of the upper airway affect the physiology of the lower airways during exercise? How does the physiology of the lower airway affect the clinical characterization of central airways disease during exercise? Does the behavior of the larynx change in clinically important ways in response to extrinsic inflammatory triggers or intrinsic distal disease? Can the characterization of the relatively well-understood lower airways lead to early identification of dysfunction in other airway sectors? Does the molecular dysregulation that causes a specific asthma endotype affect all airway sectors in ways that will change our approach to treatment of that endotype in the future? These are only a few of the questions to answer related to biologic and physiologic coupling across the airway. More broadly, can we use the experience of asthma research, which has led to a model of distinct phenotypes and precision care, guide research about other dysfunction of other airway sectors, which may also be final common pathways to constellations of phenomena?

SUMMARY

This is an exciting time in the study of interactions between exercise and the airway. It is now clear that asthma and EIB do not explain many of the symptoms attributable to the airway in exercise, with nasal disease, EILO, and EDAC contributing in select populations. Our improved understanding of these more recently appreciated conditions will continue to improve the precision of patient care moving forward.

ACKNOWLEDGMENTS

The editors thank all of the individual contributors for their diligent work in summarizing the fields featured in this issue. Dr J.T. Olin would also like to thank his wife and children for accommodating the effort required to produce this issue. He also thanks many of his previous and current in mentors for their guidance, including Jeff Davidson, Jeff Wagener, Frank Accurso, Lynn Taussig, Dan Cooper, Stan Szefler, and Bruce Bender. Dr J.H. Hull would like to acknowledge his daughters Isobel and Chloe for their support.

REFERENCES

1. Haskell WL, Lee IM, Pate RR, et al. Physical activity and public health: updated recommendation for adults from the American College of Sports Medicine and the American Heart Association. Circulation 2007;116(9):1081–93.

2. Ghory JE. Exercise and asthma: overview and clinical impact. Pediatrics 1975; 56(5 pt-2 suppl):844–6.
3. Walker A, Surda P, Rossiter M, et al. Nasal function and dysfunction in exercise. J Laryngol Otol 2016;130(5):431–4.
4. Roksund OD, Heimdal JH, Clemm H, et al. Exercise inducible laryngeal obstruction: diagnostics and management. Paediatr Respir Rev 2017;21:86–94.
5. Murgu S, Stoy S. Excessive dynamic airway collapse: a standalone cause of exertional dyspnea? Ann Am Thorac Soc 2016;13(9):1437–9.
6. Spence L, Brown WJ, Pyne DB, et al. Incidence, etiology, and symptomatology of upper respiratory illness in elite athletes. Med Sci Sports Exerc 2007;39(4): 577–86.
7. Lakin RC, Metzger WJ, Haughey BH. Upper airway obstruction presenting as exercise-induced asthma. Chest 1984;86(3):499–501.
8. Christensen PM, Thomsen SF, Rasmussen N, et al. Exercise-induced laryngeal obstructions: prevalence and symptoms in the general public. Eur Arch Otorhinolaryngol 2011;268(9):1313–9.
9. Johansson H, Norlander K, Berglund L, et al. Prevalence of exercise-induced bronchoconstriction and exercise-induced laryngeal obstruction in a general adolescent population. Thorax 2015;70(1):57–63.
10. Dunglison RD. The practice of medicine. Philadelphia: Lea and Blanchard; 1842.
11. Patterson R, Schatz M, Horton M. Munchausen's stridor: non-organic laryngeal obstruction. Clin Allergy 1974;4(3):307–10.
12. Christopher KL, Wood RP, Eckert RC, et al. Vocal-cord dysfunction presenting as asthma. N Engl J Med 1983;308(26):1566–70.
13. Olin JT, Clary MS, Fan EM, et al. Continuous laryngoscopy quantitates laryngeal behaviour in exercise and recovery. Eur Respir J 2016;48(4):1192–200.
14. Heimdal JH, Roksund OD, Halvorsen T, et al. Continuous laryngoscopy exercise test: a method for visualizing laryngeal dysfunction during exercise. Laryngoscope 2006;116:52–7.
15. Marcinow AM, Thompson J, Chiang T, et al. Paradoxical vocal fold motion disorder in the elite athlete: experience at a large division I university. Laryngoscope 2014;124(6):1425–30.
16. Olin JT, Deardorff EH, Fan EM, et al. Therapeutic laryngoscopy during exercise: a novel non-surgical therapy for refractory EILO. Pediatr Pulmonol 2017;52(6): 813–9.
17. Maat RC, Roksund OD, Olofsson J, et al. Surgical treatment of exercise-induced laryngeal dysfunction. Eur Arch Otorhinolaryngol 2007;264(4):401–7.
18. Norlander K, Johansson H, Jansson C, et al. Surgical treatment is effective in severe cases of exercise-induced laryngeal obstruction: a follow-up study. Acta Otolaryngol 2015;135(11):1152–9.
19. Weinstein DJ, Hull JE, Ritchie BL, et al. Exercise-associated excessive dynamic airway collapse in military personnel. Ann Am Thorac Soc 2016;13(9):1476–82.
20. Parsons JP, Hallstrand TS, Mastronarde JG, et al. An official American Thoracic Society clinical practice guideline: exercise-induced bronchoconstriction. Am J Respir Crit Care Med 2013;187(9):1016–27.
21. Weiler JM, Layton T, Hunt M. Asthma in United States Olympic athletes who participated in the 1996 summer games. J Allergy Clin Immunol 1998;102(5): 722–6.
22. Anderson SD, Daviskas E. The mechanism of exercise-induced asthma is.... J Allergy Clin Immunol 2000;106(3):453–9.

23. McFadden ER Jr. Hypothesis: exercise-induced asthma as a vascular phenomenon. Lancet 1990;335(8694):880–3.
24. Hull JH, Ansley L, Price OJ, et al. Eucapnic voluntary hyperpnea: gold standard for diagnosing exercise-induced bronchoconstriction in athletes? Sports Med 2016;46(8):1083–93.
25. Weiler JM, Brannan JD, Randolph CC, et al. Exercise-induced bronchoconstriction update-2016. J Allergy Clin Immunol 2016;138(5):1292–5.e36.

Moving?

Make sure your subscription moves with you!

To notify us of your new address, find your **Clinics Account Number** (located on your mailing label above your name), and contact customer service at:

Email: journalscustomerservice-usa@elsevier.com

800-654-2452 (subscribers in the U.S. & Canada)
314-447-8871 (subscribers outside of the U.S. & Canada)

Fax number: 314-447-8029

Elsevier Health Sciences Division
Subscription Customer Service
3251 Riverport Lane
Maryland Heights, MO 63043

*To ensure uninterrupted delivery of your subscription, please notify us at least 4 weeks in advance of move.

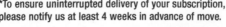

Printed and bound by CPI Group (UK) Ltd, Croydon, CR0 4YY

07/10/2024

01040504-0019